THE BIRTH PARTNER

THE
BIRTH
PARTNER

*Everything
You Need to Know
to Help a Woman
Through Childbirth*

Second Edition

Penny Simkin, P.T.

THE HARVARD COMMON PRESS
BOSTON, MASSACHUSETTS

The Harvard Common Press
535 Albany Street
Boston, Massachusetts 02118

Printed in the United States of America

Printed on acid-free paper

Library of Congress Cataloging-in-Publication Data

Simkin, Penny
        The birth partner : everything you need to know to help
a woman through childbirth / Penny Simkin.—2nd ed.
            p. cm.
        Includes bibliographical references and index
        ISBN 1-55832-195-0 (pbk. : alk. paper)
        ISBN 1-55832-193-4 (hardcover : alk. paper)
        1. Pregnancy. 2. Natural childbirth. 3. Labor
(Obstetrics)—Complications. 4. Childbirth. I. Title.

RG525.S5829 2001
618.2—dc21   00-143873

Photographs by Artemis

Drawings by Childbirth Graphics,
Faith Cogswell, and Shanna Dela Cruz

Cover design by Jackie Schuman

Special bulk-order discounts are available on this and other
Harvard Common Press books. Companies and organizations
may purchase books for premiums or resale, or may arrange a
custom edition, by contacting the Marketing Director at the
address above.

10 9 8 7 6 5 4 3 2 1

This book is dedicated . . .

To the thousands of expectant mothers and fathers who have taught me so much while I have taught them;

To the hundreds of women and their loving partners whom I have been privileged to assist during labor;

To my seven grandchildren, whose births I have attended in the role of proud grandmother;

To my four grown children, to whom I could not feel closer and of whom I could not be more proud, and to their spouses, who enrich my life;

And lastly but especially to Peter, my husband, father of our children, and my beloved partner for over four decades.

CONTENTS

ACKNOWLEDGMENTS

I have had my share of support throughout the process of revising this book. Jan Dowers, Brenda Sutherland Field, and Cinda Weber have gone far beyond the call of duty in helping me prepare the extensive revisions, helping keep my schedule clear for writing, running my office, conducting library searches, and retrieving published papers for this update. My colleagues and co-authors of *Pregnancy, Childbirth, and the Newborn*, Ann Keppler and Janet Whalley, have spent countless hours with me, sharing their extensive expertise and providing a helpful sounding board for me on many challenging matters relating to childbearing. My friend and colleague Sandy Szalay has inspired me with her dedication and commitment to young families, and with her generosity in providing them (especially my daughters' families) with advice and concrete support. Linda Ziedrich, my editor, has been extremely patient and helpful. Special thanks go to Ruth Ancheta, with whom I co-authored *The Labor Progress Handbook* and who has generously shared many of her illustrations from that book, and to Shanna Dela Cruz, who prepared most of the new illustrations. I also want to thank John Kennell, Marshall Klaus, and Phyllis Klaus, dear friends whose thoughtful insights and groundbreaking work on labor support have deepened my understanding. Finally, I want to thank my husband, Peter, who has been my patient and accepting partner throughout the labor and birth of this book.

Introduction

Congratulations! You are to be a birth partner. You have the privilege and responsibility of accompanying a woman through one of the truly unforgettable events of her life—the birth of her baby. If it is also your baby, this birth is even more significant to you. If you love the woman, as her husband, lover, friend, mother, or other relative, this birth and the woman's experience of it mean a great deal to you. Even if you hardly know the woman—if you are, for example, a nurse, a childbirth educator, a doula, or a student of nursing, midwifery, or medicine—you still recognize how important this birth and baby are to her, and you want to help her to have a positive and gratifying experience.

A woman never forgets her experiences in giving birth. And she will never forget you and how you helped her.

Although I have written this book *to* you, I have written it *for* her. My wishes for every pregnant woman are that she and her baby remain safe and healthy, and that she feel nurtured and fulfilled as she gives birth. A team of people will help her to give birth safely and with satisfaction: her caregivers (midwife, physician, or both), one or more nurses, and her birth partner(s). Your main role as her birth partner is to help her have the kind of birth she desires. And the purpose of this book is to help you help her. Having given birth myself to four children, having been present at the births of my seven grandchildren, having provided labor support for numerous women, and having spent more than thirty years teaching and learning from thousands of women and their partners, I am ready to share what I know with you.

In helping to create a fulfilling memory for your partner, you do the same for yourself. Helping a woman through childbirth and witnessing the birth of a baby rank among the high points of life.

The Language of Childbirth

As you will soon discover, there are many unfamiliar concepts and a whole new language related to pregnancy and birth. It may seem confusing at first, but you will want to understand these terms in order to communicate with nurses, caregivers (midwives and doctors), and others who are knowledgeable about the subject. To help you, I have used familiar descriptive words along with the technical terms used by professionals.

As you become more familiar with the new vocabulary, you will become more comfortable with it.

How to Use This Book

The Birth Partner is intended to be useful both as a guide to prepare you in advance for your role as birth partner and also as a quick reference during labor. Try to read the entire book before the mother goes into labor. Then, if there is time, you may want to review parts of it during labor.

But there may also be times during labor when you need immediate help and want to find something quickly in this book. Anticipating which information you may need on the spot, I have indicated certain sections by darkening the page edges. Fan the pages of the book and find those with dark edges. Their titles are listed right on the edge for quick reference. These sections are as follows:

Part One
BEFORE
THE BIRTH

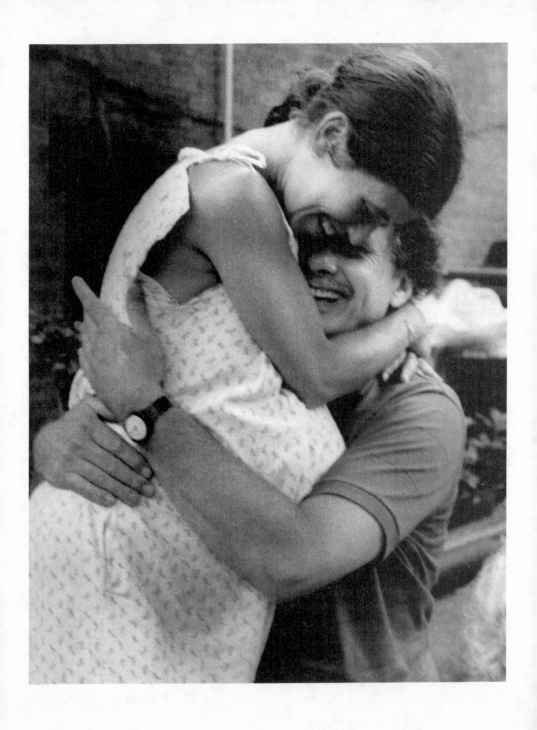

THE BIRTH PARTNER'S ROLE BEGINS BEFORE THE mother is actually in labor. During the last few weeks of her pregnancy, you can learn about labor, encourage her to continue good health habits, help her with last-minute preparations for the baby and for labor itself, and figure out the role you will play as her birth partner.

This is also the time for her to make many important decisions about the birth and to discuss them with her caregiver. If you attend childbirth classes and go to her prenatal checkups, you will not only become informed, but you will also become more comfortable in your role. Together, you will discover many important things, such as what her doctor or midwife is like, the options available in the care of mother and baby, and practical details. You can also get advice and reassurance about anything that is causing anxiety or uncertainty for either or both of you.

During these last weeks, you can prepare for your role through introspection, discussions with the pregnant mother, and helping her to gather information and practice comfort measures.

1
The Last Few Weeks
of Pregnancy

*E*arly in pregnancy, it seems that nine months is forever and that there is plenty of time to do everything that has to be done. It is all too easy, especially for busy people, to postpone "getting into" the pregnancy. Now, suddenly, the baby is almost due. Time has flown by. As the mother's birth partner, you realize she is counting on you to help her through childbirth. Do you feel ready? Can you help her? What do you know about labor? Do you know what to do when? What should you do now to get ready for the baby?

It is not too late to learn and do what needs to be done. But you had better start right away—a few weeks before the due date is truly the "last minute," especially since many babies arrive early. This first chapter is basically a checklist of things you should do before labor starts to help ensure that you will work well with the mother during the labor and birth. Also included are suggestions about how you can help prepare beforehand for the baby's arrival.

What Kind of Birth Partner Will You Be?

Birth partners come in all shapes and sizes, and they help the laboring woman in any number of ways. Most often the birth partner is the baby's father and the mother's husband or lover. The birth partner may instead be the woman's mother, sister, or friend. Or the birth partner may be the mother's lesbian lover, who will become the baby's co-parent. The role played by the birth partner varies according to many personal factors and the nature of the partner's relationship with the mother.

What role will you play? What role does the woman want you to play? How much effort do you and she want to expend learning about childbirth and practicing comfort measures? How actively does she want to participate in decision making, in coping with the pain, in helping the labor to progress well, and in delivering her baby? Does she prefer to have a more natural birth or a more medical birth?

If she wants a natural birth, she should acquire a basic understanding of childbirth, learn many techniques for coping with pain, and plan realistically for the challenges of labor. She must believe she is capable of giving birth vaginally and dealing with the stress and pain, with help and guidance from her medical team and her support team (along with the good fortune of a normal labor). She prefers to rely more on herself and her support team and less on drugs and procedures to get through labor and delivery her baby. If she wants a more medical birth, she will rely heavily on her doctor or midwife to make decisions, to use drugs and procedures to control the progress and pain of labor, and to deliver her baby. Neither preference is right or wrong, but your role as birth partner is affected by her approach to labor and birth and your comfort with her choices. Does she have thoughts about what she will want and need from you? Do you feel able and eager to help her as she wishes?

All these questions may seem impossible to answer right now. But keep them in mind as you read this book, and start discussing them with the mother. Start imagining her in labor, and the challenges you may face as her birth partner.

HOW WILL YOU FEEL?

For a realistic idea of the situations and feelings you may encounter as a birth partner, ask yourself these questions:

How will I feel when

She asks me to take time off to go to prenatal appointments with her?

She tells me that we are signed up for 12 to 18 hours of childbirth classes?

She asks me to read this book or others?

During prelabor or early labor, she wakes up moaning every 15 to 20 minutes during the night, and I am very tired?

She does not accept my suggestions for relaxation or coping?

I get tired or hungry, but she needs my help with every contraction?

The nurse is annoying or upsetting her?

She expresses discouragement ("This is so hard," "I can't keep on," "How much longer?" "Don't make me do this")?

She clings to me and says, "Help me"?

She vomits or needs to vomit?

She is in pain and begins to cry, grimace, and tense her muscles?

She criticizes me ("Not like that," "Don't touch me," "Don't breathe in my face," "Don't leave me")?

She tells me, "I want an epidural"?

She needs me to press hard on her back with every contraction, until my arms ache?

We are told that a cesarean will be necessary?

Her caregiver says, "Look here! The baby's head is starting to come"?

The baby slides out, wrinkled, soaking wet, streaked with blood, and crying?

I am asked if I want to cut the cord?

The little squirming, bundled baby is handed to me to hold and cuddle?

The new mother looks at me and says, "I couldn't have done it without you"?

Use the exercise "How Will You Feel" as a reality check. Reading this book will prepare you for such situations and help you plan good strategies to handle them. By the time labor begins, you should have a much clearer picture of yourself as birth partner.

Getting Ready for Labor

If you haven't already done the things described in the following pages, try to get them done a few weeks before the due date, or at least before labor starts.

Visit the Mother's Caregiver (Doctor or Midwife)

If you have not yet met the mother's caregiver, this visit may be more important than you think, for both the caregiver and yourselves. Even a brief meeting helps establish to the caregiver that you are an important person in the mother's life. Although a substitute caregiver may be present at the birth, this meeting provides you with an opportunity to ask your own questions and to play a more active role.

Visit the Hospital

Take a tour of the hospital maternity area—birthing rooms, nursery, and postpartum rooms. You can find out when tours are available by calling the hospital. Sometimes a tour is included in childbirth classes.

On the way to the tour, figure out your route to the hospital, how long it takes to get there, and which entrances to use during the day and at night (you may use the main entrance during the day and the emergency entrance at night).

If the mother is planning to give birth at home or in a birth center, be sure to visit the backup hospital so that you won't be confused if a transfer becomes necessary.

Preregister at the Hospital

Preregistering involves obtaining, reading, and signing pre-admission forms and a medical consent form. By registering in advance, you save time and avoid confusion when the mother is in labor.

Consider Arranging for a Doula to Help You Both During Labor

One of the most positive recent developments in maternity care from the point of view of the parents is the addition of the doula to guide and support women and their partners through labor and birth. A doula is trained and experienced in providing emotional support, physical comfort, and nonclinical advice. She draws on her knowledge of and experience with birth as she reassures, encourages and empathizes with the mother. A doula cannot and does not try to take over the role of the birth partner, who knows the mother better and loves her as no one else does. But there are times when a woman needs more than one helper in labor.

Numerous studies have examined the effects of doulas' attendance at births. In very "high-tech" hospitals with high cesarean rates, women attended by doulas have had fewer cesareans. And women attended by doulas in various birth settings have described easier postpartum emotional and physical adjustments than have other mothers.

Besides helping the mother, a doula can help you, in numerous ways:

- She can guide you in applying what you learned in childbirth class to the more stressful and unpredictable labor situation.
- She can spell you so that you can get a meal, a short nap, or just a break during a long or all-night labor.
- She can bring the mother beverages, hot packs, or ice, so that you do not have to leave her side to do so.
- She can help you understand what the mother might be feeling and interpret the signs of labor progress to you.
- If you do not feel comfortable being the mother's only constant source of support, the doula can help you to participate more comfortably by making sure the mother's needs are met.
- While getting to know the two of you before the birth, the doula can discover your priorities, fears, and concerns and help you develop strategies to deal with them.

One father described a doula this way: "She was like my big sister—ready, willing, and able to help me do the best job I could. She showed me how to rub Mary's back, reminded us to try the lunge [see page 112], and got me a bagel when I was really hungry. She kept encouraging us. She seemed so confident. A lot of the time both she and I were helping Mary. I was holding her during the contractions, and our doula was pressing on Mary's back and helping her breathe. Our doula even gave me a shoulder rub in the middle of the night. Without her, the birth wouldn't have been so great for both Mary and me. The doula helped me do a better job."

To locate a doula, contact Doulas of North America (see "Recommended Resources").

Be Sure the Mother Can Always Reach You by Phone

If necessary, rent a pager—check the Yellow Pages under "paging systems"—or carry a cell phone, and keep it turned on (the hospital may require that you turn it off when you arrive). If your job takes you far away, plan to have someone else available when you are not.

Review What You Learned in Childbirth Classes

If you have taken classes, review your handouts and notes. Gather those materials that you might want to refer to during labor—lists, suggestions, questionnaires, information about the hospital's services, and copies of the mother's Birth Plan.

Gather the Necessary Supplies

What do you pack for the hospital? What do you need for a home birth? The following lists should help.

Supplies to Take to the Hospital. From this list, select only those items that you and the mother feel will be helpful. Try to pack as many of these things in advance as possible.

- *For the mother during labor:*
    Oil or cornstarch for massage
    Lip balm

Toothbrush and toothpaste

Hairbrush and comb

Her own gown and robe if she prefers them to hospital clothes

Rolling pin, massage device, or hot or cold pack for pressure, heat, or cold on her lower back

Ponytail holder to keep long hair off her face

Warm socks and slippers

Compact discs or tapes of favorite relaxing music, and a player (if one is not available in the hospital)

Personal comfort items (pillow, flowers, pictures)

Favorite juice, frozen juice bars, or an electrolyte-balanced beverage (such as Gatorade) in a cooler (hospitals provide some juices)

- *For the birth partner:*

    Copy of the Birth Plan (see page 26)

    Watch with a second hand

    Grooming supplies (toothbrush, breath mints, deodorant, shaver)

    Food for snacks, such as sandwiches, fruit, cheese and crackers, beverages (consider what they will do to your breath)

    Sweater

    Change of clothes

    Slippers

    Swimsuit, so you can accompany the mother in the shower or bath

    Paper and pencil

    This book

    Reading materials or handwork, for slow times when the mother does not need your help

    Phone numbers of people to call during or after labor

    Telephone credit card

    Camera (still or video), film or videotape, batteries, audio tape and recorder

- *For the mother during the postpartum period:*

    Gowns that open in front for breastfeeding, unless she prefers hospital gowns

    Robe and slippers

SUPPLIES TO TAKE TO THE HOSPITAL

Cosmetics and toilet articles
Tasty snack foods, such as fruit, nuts, cheese and crackers
Nursing bras
Money for incidentals
Going-home clothing

- *For the baby:*
    Clothing: diapers, waterproof pants, undershirt or onesie, gown or stretch suit, receiving blanket, outer clothing (hat, warm clothing), crib-sized blanket
    Car seat, properly installed (have it checked by an auto dealer, or call the Auto Safety Hotline at (800) 424-9393 for information)

- *For the trip to the hospital:*
    A full tank of gas
    A blanket and pillow in the car

Supplies for a Home Birth. Look over the preceding lists for ideas about what to have at home. In addition, consider the following.

- *Birthing supplies* (ask the midwife for a list, or go over this one with her):
    Disposable waterproof underpads (Chux pads)
    Sterile 4-by-4-inch gauze pads
    K-Y jelly
    Bulb syringe
    Cord clamps
    Squeeze bottle to cleanse perineum
    Waterproof mattress cover (a shower curtain will do)
    Wet, folded washcloths placed in plastic bags and frozen
    Thermometer
    Basin for the placenta
    Washcloths and hand towels
    At least two sets of clean bed sheets
    Flexible straws
    Trash bags
    Birthing tub (available for rent)

- *Other supplies—*
    Long, maternity-sized sanitary pads
    Hat for the baby

Food for the birthing team during labor
Food and drink for a birth celebration
A map to your home, for the midwife and doula

For a home birth, you will want to make some other preparations at the last minute: Turn up the water heater, and be sure everyone in the household knows that you have done so. Clean and organize the house. Make the bed with fresh linens (that you don't mind getting stained) by putting a cotton sheet over the mattress, a waterproof mattress cover or plastic sheet over the cotton sheet, and another cotton sheet over the waterproof cover or sheet. (During labor and birth, the top sheet may become stained and wet. After the birth, the top sheet and waterproof sheet can be quickly removed, and the other clean sheet will be already in place.) In case of transfer to a hospital, know the way to the backup hospital, have plenty of gas in your car's tank, and include in the Birth Plan the mother's preferences in case of transfer (see "Review the Mother's Birth Plan," page 26).

Encourage the Mother to Drink Plenty of Fluids

During pregnancy, the mother should drink at least two quarts of liquid a day—water, fruit juices, clear soups. This helps support her increased fluid needs.

Help Her Switch to a High-Carbohydrate Diet

Just as an endurance athlete benefits from "carbo-loading" for a few days before an athletic event, a pregnant woman may benefit from a high-carbohydrate (high-starch) diet at the end of pregnancy in preparation for her "event"—labor.

Benefits of a High-Carbohydrate Diet. A diet high in starchy foods has been shown to increase the amount of glycogen stored in muscle. During muscular exertion (such as uterine contractions during labor), the glycogen is converted to glucose, the muscle's energy source. If the body's glycogen stores are depleted, then fat is converted into glycogen. Fat conversion, however, does not work as well as glycogen conversion. As fat is used to provide energy, byproducts called ketone bodies accumulate in the blood, causing ketosis, a condition that can slow labor or, if the buildup is great, even cause fetal distress. If a laboring woman develops ketosis, intravenous fluids containing dextrose (sugar) may be given to provide energy and thus correct the ketosis. A high-carbohydrate diet late in pregnancy may provide enough glycogen to prevent ketosis.

Foods She Should Eat. During the last few days of pregnancy, the mother should shift toward carbohydrates as her major source of calories. The recommendation for athletes is 60 to 65 percent of caloric intake as carbohydates. The following foods help build glycogen stores in muscle: bread, crackers, cereal, waffles, pancakes, corn, pasta, potatoes, rice, and fresh fruit. Protein and fat should make up a smaller proportion of her diet than carbohydrates. Small amounts of milk or cheese, meat, fish, tofu, lentils, and very small amounts of butter, margarine, and oil can be added to make the starchy foods more tasty. In addition, she should not ignore fresh vegetables.

In early labor, and especially in the slow-to-start labor (page 137), the mother should drink plenty of water, caffeine-free tea, fruit juice, or sports beverages. In addition, she should eat easily digested, high-carbohydrate, starchy foods. These can help prevent undue fatigue.

Caution: If she has diabetes, she should follow the dietary guidelines she has been given by her caregiver.

Encourage Her to Exercise

Regular exercise such as walking or swimming will help to maintain the mother's general fitness. In addition, a few special exercises are particularly helpful during late pregnancy and labor. These are squatting, the pelvic rock on hands and knees, and the Kegel (pelvic-floor contraction) exercise. Encourage the mother to do these every day.

Squatting. Squatting may be very useful in helping the baby come down during the birthing stage (see page 114), but, because it is not a customary position for Westerners, the mother may need to get used to it before labor begins.

Wearing loose clothing, she should stand with her feet wide enough apart that she can keep her heels on the floor as she

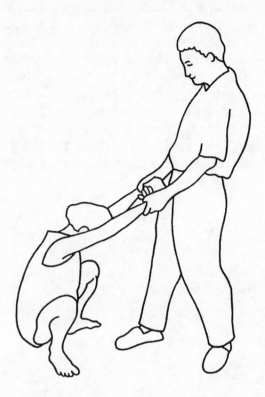

squats. Then she lowers herself into a squatting position. It is not necessary that she have perfect balance. She can hold onto you, the arm of a couch, or doorknobs on either side of a door. She can also rest her back against a wall or against you, if you sit behind her. Once squatting, she should remain in the position (without bouncing) for up to 1 minute (she might begin with 20 seconds and gradually increase the time). Then she rises to standing. If she does 10 squats a day, she will rapidly become accustomed to the position.

If her insteps roll in, she can correct this by placing each heel on a book (1 to 2 inches thick). This way she still has her weight on her heels while relieving pressure on her insteps.

A woman should *not* practice squatting if it causes her undue or lasting pain. She should also refrain from this exercise if she has hip, knee, or ankle problems that could be worsened by squatting.

Pelvic Rock on Hands and Knees. During pregnancy, this exercise helps strengthen abdominal muscles, relieve low back pain, improve circulation in the lower half of the body, and position the baby in the favorable OA (occiput anterior) position (see page 44). During labor it helps relieve back pain and rotate the baby.

The mother should get down on her hands and knees, and make herself "square"; that is, her thighs and arms should be perpendicular to the floor and her back straight, not sagging. Then she tucks her "tail" under, feeling the tightening of her abdominal muscles and some stretching and arching in her low back. She holds the position for ten seconds, then returns to the original position. (This exercise is easy to do while reading the newspaper!) If she practices prenatal yoga, she will recognize this as similar to the "cat-cow" exercise. She should repeat the pelvic rock 10 times a day.

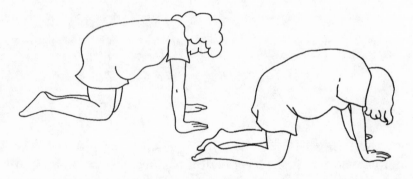

The Kegel (Pelvic Floor Contraction) Exercise. This is the most important of the three exercises to a woman's lifelong general health, because it strengthens muscles that support the pelvic organs and that are vital to sexual pleasure. During childbirth, good tone in these muscles helps the baby rotate and descend. The mother's ability to relax these muscles in the second stage as she pushes her baby down the birth canal will greatly assist the birth.

There are two components of the Kegel exercise—toning and bulging.

1. *Pelvic floor toning.* The mother contracts the muscles of her pelvic floor as she might when she is trying to keep from urinating or stopping the flow of urine once it has begun. She

can do some quick contractions ("flicks") and hold others for up to 30 seconds. She will find that the longer holds ("super-Kegels") are difficult to maintain; these muscle fibers seem to fatigue fairly quickly, even in women with good tone. If the contraction seems to disappear or fade, even when she has not consciously let go, she should simply renew it by tightening again. She lets go and rests after 20 to 30 seconds, or sooner if she is unable to keep renewing the contraction. She should try not to contract muscles in her legs, buttocks, or abdomen, or to hold her breath while doing the exercise.

She should try to do super-Kegels at least 10 times a day. You can remind her to do them while riding in the car or bus, waiting in line, or talking on the telephone. It may be easiest for her to do one or two while washing her hands after using the toilet.

2. *Pelvic floor bulging.* This exercise is a rehearsal for "letting go" during the birthing stage as the baby stretches the vagina and comes out. The mother can help the baby emerge by relaxing her pelvic floor muscles, rather than tensing or tightening them. This is how she should practice:

After doing a super-Kegel, she lets go of the contraction and then consciously bulges her pelvic floor by holding her breath and gently straining as she would to press out the last few drops of urine or a bowel movement. She then teaches herself to bulge her pelvic floor while exhaling. She should always conclude a bulging exercise by contracting, then relaxing the pelvic floor. One or two of these exercises a day are probably enough to prepare her for the birth.

A woman should do the pelvic floor toning exercise all her life. The bulging exercise is important for only a few weeks before birth.

You Should Exercise, Too

Labor can be physically demanding for you as well as for the mother. A strong partner is invaluable in helping the mother change and maintain certain positions (see pages 112), and in providing steady pressure on her low back or hips to relieve back pain (see page 127). Furthermore, you will need physical stamina to remain awake and on your feet for hours. If you are not in very good shape, you might want to begin some strength training, particularly for your arms, chest, shoulders, and back.

Push-ups, sit-ups, back exercises, and weight training will improve your strength. See "Recommended Resources" for a list of books on strength building.

Use Prenatal Perineal Massage

As scientific studies have confirmed, regular massage of the inside of a woman's perineum (the area between the vagina and the anus) in late pregnancy helps prepare the perineum to stretch adequately during the birth. Prenatal perineal massage can reduce the need for an episiotomy (a surgical incision to enlarge the vagina, done just before the birth), and reduces the likelihood that the mother's tissues will spontaneously tear during birth. Prenatal perineal massage lets the expectant mother experience sensations that are similar to those she will feel as the baby emerges, and it gives her a chance to practice relaxing her perineum as she should during delivery.

I advise pregnant women in my classes to use perineal massage for four to six weeks before their due date. Frankly, some women find the massage distasteful and decide not to do it; others find it pleasurable or sexually stimulating, which is a bonus. Most who do it regularly find it very beneficial.

Caution: If vaginitis, a herpes sore, or another vaginal problem exists, perineal massage could worsen or spread the condition and should not be done until the problem goes away.

Instructions for Perineal Massage. Either you or the expectant mother herself can do the massage. It is easier for her to have you do it.

These directions are for you:

1. Be sure your fingernails are short. Wash your hands before beginning. If you have rough skin on your fingers that might scratch her, wear disposable rubber gloves.

2. Have the mother make herself comfortable in a semi-sitting position, with her legs bent and relaxed.

3. Lubricate your fingers well with wheat-germ oil or other vegetable oil, or with water-soluble jelly. Do not use baby oil, mineral oil, or petroleum jelly, as they tend to dry the tissue; vegetable oils are better absorbed. To avoid contaminating the oil, do not dip your fingers in it; instead, squirt the oil over your fingers.

4. Use your index fingers. Start with one and progress to two. Place your fingers well inside the expectant mother's vagina (up to the second knuckle); rotate them in opposite directions upward along the sides and back to the center while pulling outward gently.

5. Tell the expectant mother to concentrate on relaxing her perineum as she feels the pressure. As she becomes more comfortable with the massage, increase the pressure just enough to make the perineum begin to sting from the stretching.

6. Continue the massage for about 3 minutes. In the beginning the tissue will feel tight, but with time and repeated massages it will relax and stretch.

7. Ask your caregiver or your childbirth educator to answer any questions you may have after trying the massage.

Perineal massage stretches the vaginal tissue, the muscles surrounding the vagina, and the skin of the perineum. After doing the massage three or four days in a row, you will probably find that the mother clearly tolerates the stretching better than at first, and that you have to increase the pressure to cause stinging. This is a good sign. The mother will still feel a stinging sensation as the baby's head is being born, but by then she will know how to relax despite the stinging.

Consider Keeping Track of Fetal Movements

Fetal movement counting is a test of the baby's well-being that sometimes detects a problem in time to prevent serious harm. Although most babies have no problems in the uterus, some do, and a major purpose of maternity care is to prevent, detect, or treat such problems.

An active baby is a healthy baby. If a baby is not doing well or is not getting enough oxygen or nourishment from his mother via the placenta, he will slow his movements to conserve energy. There is usually a period of decreasing movement—enough time to act—before the baby is in serious trouble.

The mother can provide an accurate daily account of fetal movements. This information can help the caregiver decide whether other tests of fetal well-being are necessary or whether to deliver the baby early. The mother is most likely to assess fetal movements correctly if she sets aside a period of time each day and keeps a written record of the time it takes to record 10 fetal movements. Such a record is more accurate than the mother's informal impressions, which are influenced by how busy or distracted she is at any particular time.

Some caregivers ask all their pregnant clients to keep a daily or every-other-day record of fetal movements from about the thirty-second week of pregnancy. Others ask only those clients who are at high risk for fetal problems. Many women find fetal movement counting to be fun and interesting. Not only do they gather helpful information, but they enjoy the time spent focusing on their babies. They learn about different types of movements, about their babies' sleep and wake cycles, and about other things. Other women find fetal movement counting makes them worry; they feel they are just waiting for something to go wrong.

FETAL MOVEMENT COUNTS

Date	Starting time	Movements	Time of tenth movement	Time elapsed
7/1/01	8:45 a.m.	╫╫╫ ╫╫╫	9:05 a.m.	20 min.

If the mother decides to count fetal movements, do it with her, at least some of the time. You can learn a lot about the baby too, and you can also support the mother if she finds it stressful.

There are several ways to do fetal movement counting. The "Count-to-Ten" method, which follows, is simple and can be begun at any time in late pregnancy.

How to Count Fetal Movements. It is most helpful if the mother counts the baby's movements every day (if she skips a day now and then, she should simply resume counting the next day). She can begin any time after the thirty-second week of pregnancy. It makes sense to begin counting when the baby is awake and active. Babies tend to be most active right after meals.

The mother writes down the time she starts counting. A movement may be a short kick or wiggle, or a long, continuous squirming. She waits for a pause in activity, and then counts it as one movement. The pause may last only a few seconds or, if the baby falls asleep, more than an hour. Hiccups do not count as movements.

When the mother has counted 10 fetal movements, she writes down the time when the tenth movement occurred, and figures how long it took to count 10 fetal movements. If she has not felt 10 movements in 12 hours, she should call her caregiver to report this information. In addition, if she finds the baby seems to be "slowing down"—that is, taking longer and longer over a period of several days to complete 10 movements, she should report this finding as well.

Prepare Other Children for the Birth

Things go more smoothly if siblings are prepared in advance for the arrival of a new brother or sister. It reassures children to know where their mother will be during the birth, where they will be, and who will be with them. And they will surely benefit from being included, as appropriate, in preparations for the new baby.

See "Recommended Resources" for books on the subject of children and birth.

Review the Mother's Birth Plan

So that you will really know how to help her, become familiar with the mother's written Birth Plan. The Birth Plan tells everyone involved in her care what options are important to her, what her priorities are, and how she would like to be cared for. If you are the mother's life partner (lover, husband, father of the baby) as well as her birth partner, the Birth Plan should be written by both of you. If you are not intimately involved with the mother, the Birth Plan should be hers, and you should be very familiar with it.

Although Birth Plans are most useful for births in hospitals, where the nurses (and often the caregivers) do not know the mother, it is useful for everyone, even those planning to give birth at home or in a birth center, to think through their priorities and choices. It helps if the two of you go over the plan together with her caregiver. At the least, however, be ready to ask the staff to read and follow the mother's plan, and be ready to remind her of some of her prior choices if she forgets them when she is caught up in the intense demands of labor.

The Birth Plan will be most useful if it is short and concise, but not in the form of a checklist. A sentence or brief paragraph on the relevant items below will work very well.

Keep a copy of the Birth Plan with you during labor. Use it as a guide, but be flexible and willing to accept changes in the plan if medical circumstances require it.

Discuss with the mother beforehand the following points in the Birth Plan and any other details that seem appropriate.

Introduction to the Birth Plan. The plan might begin with the following information:

- *Personal information.* What would the mother like the staff to know about her? For example, she might describe strongly held beliefs or preferences, relevant previous experiences with hospitals or health care, fears, concerns, or other information that would help the staff get to know her and treat her as a special individual.
- *Message to the staff.* Would she like to express her appreciation for any support, expertise, and assistance the staff can provide to help her have a safe and satisfying birth experience?

Labor Options. The mother can consider the following options for labor:

- *Activity in labor.* Does she want the freedom to walk, change positions, take a bath or shower, or move about in labor to promote comfort or progress? Or will she be content to remain in bed? (See "Movement and Position Changes," page 111.)
- *Food and drink.* Does she prefer to eat and drink at will, or is she comfortable with having intravenous fluids (see page 177) and sucking ice chips?
- *Fetal heart-rate monitoring.* How does she feel about continuous electronic monitoring (internal or external), intermittent monitoring, or, instead, having a nurse or caregiver listen with an ultrasound stethoscope or a regular stethoscope? (See "Electronic Fetal Monitoring" page 180.)
- *Pain medications.* Does she plan to use them? Does she want them as soon as she goes into labor, or will she try to delay them until mid- to late labor? Does she want to avoid pain medications entirely, if possible? How important is this to her? (See chapter 8, and especially the "Pain Medications Preference Scale" on page 249, for important information and pointers.)

Birth Options. The mother can consider the following options for birth:

- *Positions for second (birthing) stage.* Would the mother prefer to be free to move, and to use a variety of positions, or is she content to be semireclining or flat on her back with her legs in footrests or stirrups? (See "Positions and Movements for Labor and Birth," page 112.)
- *Pushing techniques.* Does she prefer to use the spontaneous, nondirected bearing-down technique or the prolonged breathholding and straining of directed pushing? (See "Breathing Patterns for Pushing," page 109.)
- *Perineal care.* Would she prefer to have warm compresses and other measures to avoid an episiotomy, or not? How strongly does she feel about this? Would she rather risk a tear than have an episiotomy? (See "Episiotomy," page 195.) If she has been doing perineal massage, she might say so.

After-Birth Options. The mother can consider the following options in postpartum care:

- *General preferences.* Are the usual routines for baby care acceptable? Does the mother want the staff to do most of the baby care? Or do the two of you prefer to do it? Do you want to be informed in advance of all procedures involving the baby?
- *Immediate care of the baby.* Do you and the mother have preferences regarding newborn routines (eye care, vitamin K, newborn exam, and so forth)? (See "Common Procedures in Newborn Care," page 277, and "The Next Few Days for the Baby," page 283.)
- *Contact with the baby.* Does the mother want to have her baby with her continuously? How does she feel about the baby's spending time in the nursery? Does she want the baby with her at night as well as during the day? Does she prefer to have the baby for feeding only?
- *Your presence.* Would the mother like you to stay in the hospital with her? Can you use a cot or fold-out chair and sleep there overnight?
- *Feeding.* Will the baby be breastfed or formula fed? If she is breastfeeding, how does the mother feel about the baby's being given water, sugar water, or formula? Does she want to feed the baby on cue (that is, when the baby expresses an interest? (See "Getting Started with Breastfeeding," page 301.) If the baby is to be formula fed, do the two of you want to do all the feeding yourselves or do you want to have the nurses do some of it?
- *Circumcision.* If the baby is a boy, will he be circumcised or not? (See "Circumcision" in chapter 10, page 284.)

The Unexpected. The mother should think through the possibility of such difficulties as the following:

- *Difficult labor.* Is the Birth Plan flexible enough to apply even if complications or difficulties arise during labor? (Using phrases like "as long as labor proceeds normally" or "unless medically indicated" leaves room for changes in the Birth Plan if safety becomes an issue.) If difficulties do arise, does the mother still want to be consulted before procedures are performed, or would she prefer to leave all decisions to the staff? And if labor is very long, who else can help so that you can eat, sleep, or just take a break? A relative, or a doula?

- *Transfer.* If she develops complications and has to be transferred from a birthing room or home to a hospital labor room, does she have some preferences regarding her care? For example: Does she want you, her doula, and any other support people to remain with her? Does she want the original Birth Plan to be respected, and does she want to keep whatever options are still possible? Does she want her caregivers to seek her informed consent for all procedures, as long as it is medically safe to do so?

- *Cesarean birth.* Does the mother want you and her doula to be present? Would she prefer to be awake? Would she like to see and touch the baby afterwards? Would she like you to go with the baby to the nursery after the birth, or to stay with her? (If she has a doula, the doula can stay with her while you go to the nursery.) What about postoperative sedation? Would she prefer to receive sleep or sedative medications afterwards or to accept some trembling and nausea in order to remain awake and to hold and nurse the baby? (See chapter 9.)

- *Premature or sick infant.* Would the mother prefer to be involved, or have you involved, as much as possible in the care and feeding of the baby, even if the baby is in the special-care unit? Does she want explanations of the baby's problems, the procedures to be done, and the decisions that need to be made? Does she want you to accompany the baby to a different hospital if the baby has to be transferred? Does she want to express her colostrum (the "pre-milk" her breasts make during the first two or three days after birth) and her milk to store until the baby can take it? (See pages 218-221.)

- *Stillbirth or death of the baby.* Such a tragedy leaves the parents so stunned with grief that it is almost impossible for them to make important decisions. Discuss this possibility together, and think about how you and the mother would want the situation handled. Weeks or months after the death of a baby, the things that were done (or not done) at the time will be very important. Consider some or all of the following:

An opportunity to hold and say good-bye to the baby in
   private

A chance to dress the baby

Mementos—pictures, the baby's clothing or blanket, a
   lock of hair, hand- and footprints

Help from a counselor or a member of the clergy

An opportunity to discuss the birth and the baby's problems with the doctor, midwife, nurses, and doula

An autopsy to determine the cause of death

A memorial service or funeral—an opportunity for family
   and friends to acknowledge the baby's life and death
   and to demonstrate their love, support, and sympathy
   for the parents

As difficult as it may be to face the possibility that the baby
could die, it is wise to think through this situation. I hope you
will never need to implement any of the above suggestions. If
you do, you will be glad later that you had thought about it
ahead of time, when you were calm and able to think clearly.

Personal Choices. Are there other choices that will help make
this birth experience more comfortable or memorable for the
mother and for you? Consider doing the following:

Providing her favorite music

Including others—doula, relatives, friends, interpreter (if
   needed), or children

Excluding nonessential personnel (for example, students,
   observers)

Having you assist in delivering the baby or cutting the umbilical cord

Photographing, videotaping, or audiotaping the birth

Using comfort items such as toothbrush, lip balm, cold
   packs, eyeglasses (if needed), lollipops, ice or fluids, a
   tool for backrubs, warm socks, cornstarch or oil for
   massage, and so forth

Welcoming the baby (with private time together, with
   music, or with a religious or personal ceremony)

Incorporating culturally significant customs (foods,
   bathing, contact with baby, and so forth)

Make sure you know the mother's preferences, and be sure they are included in her written Birth Plan.

Preparing for Life with the Baby

Following is a reminder list of some things to try to do before the baby is born. It is much easier to do these things before the birth than afterwards, when time and energy will be more limited. If you are the mother's life partner (husband, lover), you will want to make these preparations together. If not, you might advise her that these need to be done.

Gather the Essential Supplies for the Baby

Is everything ready for the baby? Are the necessary supplies on hand? Use the lists that follow as a guide.

- *Baby equipment*
  Car seat (install it correctly and have it checked; see page 16)
  Crib, bassinet, cradle, or baby bed that attaches to your bed

- *Bedding (minimum requirements)*
  Two or more fitted sheets (pillowcases often fit bassinette mattresses)
  Two square waterproof pads to fit under the baby's diaper area
  Two warm, crib-sized blankets or quilts
  Three receiving blankets

- *Clothing* (Buy baby clothes with room for growing—no smaller than 10- to 12-pound size. Babies usually weigh close to 10 pounds by the time they are one to two months old, if not at birth. Often babies outgrow even six-month-size clothes by the time they are two or three months old.)
  Four snap- or tie-front undershirts, or pullover undershirts that snap at the crotch
  Three one-piece coveralls (stretch suits, sleepers) or nightgowns
  Two sweaters

One hat for indoors the first few days
One hat for outdoors
One warm outfit for outdoors
Two pairs of booties
Four pinless diaper covers, plastic pants, or soakers
At least two to four dozen cloth diapers and a diaper pail, unless the mother plans to use a diaper service, or at least 80 newborn-size disposable diapers (even if she plans to use disposables, cloth diapers make great burp cloths)
Three pairs of diaper pins, if necessary
Two baby bath towels
Two washcloths

- *Health supplies*
  Blunt fingernail scissors
  Thermometer for measuring underarm temperature
  Cornstarch, for powdering diaper area
  Diaper-rash ointment
  Baby wipes

- *Supplies for breastfeeding*
  At least two well-fitting nursing bras
  Nursing pads (commercially available, or she can make her own—six layers of cotton flannel cut into rounds to fit inside her bra and sewn together)

- *Supplies for formula feeding*
  Formula
  Eight to twelve bottles with nipples and caps
  Nipple brush, for washing nipples

- *Optional paraphernalia*
  Bumper pads for crib
  Mobile (choose one with black and white or other high-contrast colors that looks interesting from below)
  Infant seat (an infant car seat can double as one of these)
  Soft front-carrier or sling (for carrying the baby with hands free)
  Stroller or carriage
  Birth ball (for sitting on and bouncing while holding the baby against your shoulder)

Baby swing
Rocking chair
Baby bathtub
Pacifiers (in case the baby needs to suck a great deal)
Breast pump (if the mother will want to express and store
  breast milk)
Intercom (if the baby will sleep beyond easy hearing range)
Tapes or records of soothing heartbeat sounds, nature
  sounds, lullabies, other music
Toys (the possibilities are endless)
Books on baby feeding, baby care, and infant development
  (see "Recommended Resources")

Choose a Caregiver or Clinic for the Baby

The baby will need a medical caregiver (pediatrician, family
doctor, nurse practitioner, naturopath, or health clinic) to provide well-baby care (routine checkups, immunizations) and to
treat illnesses if they occur. Get recommendations from friends,
the mother's childbirth educator, or her caregiver. You and the
mother can interview possible caregivers before the birth, often
without charge (when making an appointment for an interview,
ask if there will be a fee). The following are important considerations when choosing a caregiver:

- *Location of the office.* How far away is it? There is a real advantage to its being close to home. Traveling a long distance
  with a sick child can be nerve-wracking.
- *Practical considerations.* What are the caregiver's educational
  and professional qualifications? What are the fees? Is the practice covered when the caregiver is not available? By whom? At
  which hospital(s) does the caregiver have privileges?
- *Philosophy of infant health care.* What are the caregiver's
  attitudes about breastfeeding, introducing solid foods,
  circumcision, immunizations, feeding and sleeping, day care,
  and so on?
- *Personal attributes.* Does this caregiver seem kind, competent, and caring? Is this someone you and the mother like and
  could trust with the baby's health care?

Prepare a Place at Home for the Baby

Whether the baby will have a fully equipped nursery or a corner of a room, you will need to organize space for the baby—for storing clothes, for diaper changing, for sleeping, and for all the equipment that comes along with babies.

Register for Infant-Care or Parenting Classes

Suggest that the mother investigate the available classes and register for any that appeal to her. If you are also the baby's parent, take a class with her. These classes deal with child development, emotional needs of parents and infants, and common problems. Parents learn exercises, songs, and games to play with their children besides having the opportunity to share their concerns with other new parents.

Prepare Meals Ahead of Time

You may be surprised to find that simply going to the store or even figuring out what to eat can seem almost overwhelming in the first weeks after the baby arrives. So stock the kitchen with nutritious foods that are easy to prepare and eat. If a freezer is available, cook food ahead and freeze it for reheating later. Locate stores and delis where prepared dishes and nutritious convenience foods are available. See chapter 10 for more suggestions about putting together quick, nutritious meals.

Plan to Share Responsibilities

You will probably be astounded by the amount of work and time it takes to feed and care for a new baby and mother, and to keep the household running. Plan to share the baby-care responsibilities and to take over much of the housework and cooking, or make arrangements for someone else to help. Remember that a baby needs almost constant care for the first few weeks. If the new mother tries to do it all, she will get much less sleep than usual. Full-time newborn care is tiring enough, but because the mother will also be recovering from the physical demands of birth, or possibly from major surgery if she gives birth by cesarean, it may take weeks for her to recover.

Many fathers or partners use vacation time or family leave to stay at home for the first days or weeks to share the work. The baby's grandparents or other relatives can also be a great source of help, as long as the mother's relationship with them is not strained. If the mother and her parents or in-laws do not get along well, their relationship will *not* suddenly improve with the arrival of the baby. Friends can be wonderful about providing meals, running errands, doing chores. Say yes if they offer to help.

In many communities, postpartum doulas are available to help new families. They come to the home and do whatever needs to be done in the way of light housekeeping, meal preparation, and errand running. More importantly, they are very knowledgeable about newborn care and feeding, and can teach new parents a great deal. A postpartum doula also can identify problems in mother or baby and make referrals if necessary. Hiring a postpartum doula can make it possible for you both to spend time just enjoying the baby and to relax a bit or get a nap. She will probably come to your home for a few hours each day for a week or two. You should book a postpartum doula before the birth.

The services of a postpartum doula are a popular gift for distant grandparents to give their children. Many grandparents wish they could come and help, but cannot, for various reasons. If a postpartum doula is not available, a house cleaner or a teenage helper may help ease some of the burden on new parents.

On to the Next Step . . .

Once you have prepared as much as possible, enjoy yourselves as you wait for labor to begin. Photograph the expectant mother at the end of her pregnancy; enjoy some evenings out for dinner, movies, concerts, plays, visits with friends and family. Plan enjoyable activities with other children. Make these last days relaxed and enjoyable before your lives change forever.

And now that you know how to really help the expectant mother *before* labor, let's go on to the next step—how you can really help her *during* labor and birth.

Part Two
LABOR AND BIRTH

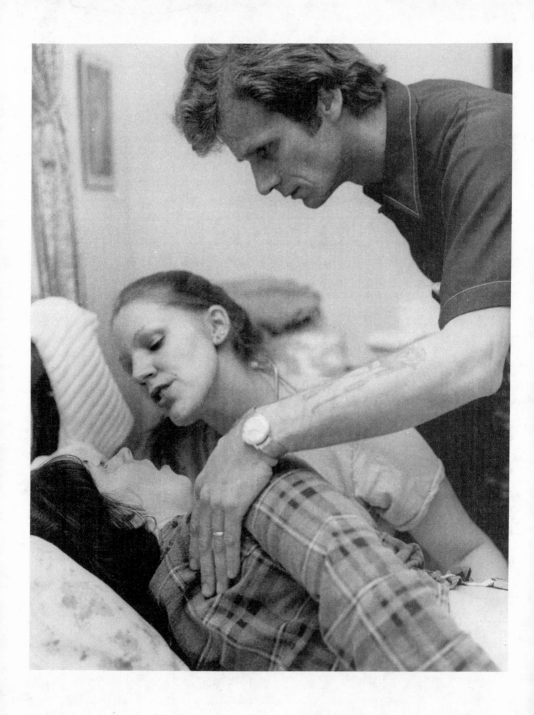

THE CLIMAX OF PREGNANCY, THE BIRTH OF A baby, is an everyday miracle—part of a day's work for the doctor, midwife, or nurse, but a deep and permanent memory for the birthing woman and those who love her and support her. Your role as the birth partner is to do as much as you can to *help make this birth experience a good memory for her*. She will never forget this birth. She will not only remember many of the events; she will remember and even relive the feelings she had. The kind of care a woman receives and the quality of the support she gets during labor make the difference in whether she looks back on her birth experience with satisfaction and fulfillment or with disappointment and sadness. This is where you come in. Being a birth partner—helping a woman through labor and birth—is clearly a challenge, but it is a challenge that people like you meet all the time.

To be a good birth partner, you need

- A bond of love or friendship with the mother and a feeling of commitment and responsibility toward her.
- Familiarity with her personal preferences and quirks, with the little things that soothe and relax her, and the things that may irritate or worry her.
- Knowledge of what to expect—the physical process of labor, the procedures and interventions commonly used during labor, and when these procedures and interventions are necessary and when they are optional.
- An understanding of the emotional side of labor—the emotional needs of women during labor and the pattern of emotions they usually experience as labor progresses.
- Practical knowledge of how to help in various situations—what to do when.
- Flexibility to adapt to the mother's changing needs during labor. This is "leading by following": how you help, and how much you help, is determined by the mother's needs and responses at the time.

If you also love the mother and the baby, you will care for them in the intimate and personal way that only a husband or

39

loved one can. The next few chapters will cover the normal birth process and will explain what happens, how the mother responds, what the caregiver does, and how you can help. They will also discuss situations that are particularly difficult for the mother and that are therefore particularly challenging for you. Read these chapters in advance, then use them as an on-the-spot guide during labor.

2
Getting into Labor

*E*veryone wonders how to tell if a woman is in labor. Even for those with vast experience, it is rarely clear exactly when labor starts. Often the mother "sneaks" into labor with unclear, on-again-off-again signs—like an orchestra tuning up before a performance. Then, over the course of many days, she gradually becomes mentally and physically ready for the coordinated effort that eventually results in the birth of the baby. Almost every woman experiences a period of uncertainty and questioning while she awaits clear signs that she is truly in labor.

As long as the two of you eventually put the pieces together, it usually doesn't matter if the mother's labor is vague at the beginning. There is almost always plenty of time, once she is clearly in labor, to get to the hospital or settle in for a home birth. Occasionally, however, a woman is caught by surprise, going into labor earlier or more suddenly than she anticipated. Because of this possibility, you will want to be able to tell the difference between the tuning up (or prelabor) and the real thing (progressing labor).

This chapter will help you both to recognize when the mother is in labor. It explains how she gets into labor both physically

and emotionally and describes the role you should play as her
birth partner.

The Labor Process

Labor is the process by which a woman gives birth to a baby.
The labor process involves the following:

1. Contractions of the uterus, the largest and strongest
muscle in the woman's body.

2. Softening (ripening), thinning (effacement), and opening
(dilation) of the cervix.

3. Breaking of the bag of waters (the membranes or amniotic
sac) that surrounds the baby, and the release of the water (amniotic fluid).

4. Rotation of the baby and molding of his or her head to fit
into the pelvis.

5. Descent of the baby out of the uterus and through the
birth canal (vagina) to the outside.

6. Birth of the placenta.

Labor usually does not begin until both mother and baby are
ready. The last weeks of pregnancy prepare the mother physically and psychologically to give birth, to breastfeed, and to
nurture a baby. During this time the baby acquires the "final
touches," preparing him or her to handle the stress of labor and
to adapt to life outside the uterus.

Occasionally babies are born prematurely, before they are
really ready. Sometimes they are born postmaturely, after
their ideal time. In these cases, babies may need special care in
the hospital.

How Long Will Labor Last?

It is impossible to predict how long any particular labor will
last. A perfectly normal labor can take between two and
twenty-four hours. In addition, some women experience prelabor contractions for a day or more before labor really begins,
that is, before the cervix begins dilating steadily.

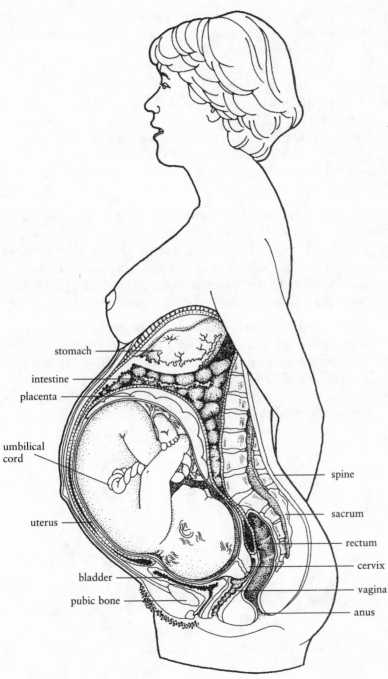

stomach

intestine

placenta

umbilical
cord

uterus

bladder

pubic bone

spine

sacrum

rectum

cervix

vagina

anus

A pregnant woman's anatomy.

Many factors influence the length of labor:

- Whether this is a first or later baby.
- The condition of the cervix (soft and thin or firm and thick) when contractions begin.
- The size of the baby, particularly the head, in relation to the size of the mother's pelvis.
- The presentation and position of the baby's head within the mother's body.
- The strength and frequency of the contractions.
- The mother's emotional state—if she is lonely, frightened, or angry she may have a longer labor than if she is confident, content, and calm.

Presentation refers to the part of the baby—top of the head (the vertex), brow, face, buttocks, feet, shoulders—that will be born first. The top of the head almost always *presents* first; problems occur in delivery if any of the others present first.

Position refers to the placement of the presenting part within the mother's pelvis. The most common positions are

- *OA* (occiput anterior): The back of the baby's head (the occiput) points toward the mother's front (anterior).
- *OT* (occiput transverse): The back of the baby's head points toward the mother's side (transverse).
- *OP* (occiput posterior): The back of the baby's head points toward the mother's back (posterior).

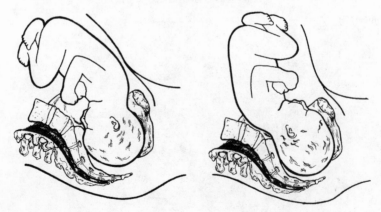

A baby in OA (occiput anterior) position (left) *and OP (occiput posterior) position* (right).

The OA and OT positions are more common than OP. When the baby is in the OP position, with the back of his head toward the mother's back, labor is sometimes prolonged, and the mother may experience intense backache.

Signs of Labor

How are you going to know when the mother is in labor? A few clues can help you recognize labor long before the birth is imminent. It is equally important, though, to be able to tell when she is not in labor. There is nothing more frustrating or disappointing for a woman than thinking she is in labor and discovering, after a trip to the caregiver, that she is not.

If you both know the signs of labor (see the table on pages 46–47) and how to interpret them, you will be more likely to react appropriately. Some of these signs are more definite than others. They are categorized as Possible Signs, Preliminary Signs, and Positive Signs.

- *Possible Signs.* Without other signs, these are not clear enough to get excited about. They may be due to something besides labor, such as indigestion, fatigue, or physical overexertion, or they may be mere "tuning up" for labor. They reassure you that the mother is moving in the right direction, but that is usually their only significance. If, however, the mother has had a rapid labor with a previous birth, she should be particularly alert to the Possible Signs to avoid being surprised by another rapid labor.
- *Preliminary Signs.* These are more important than the Possible Signs, but it could still be hours or even days before labor is really underway.
- *Positive Signs.* These are the only certain signs that the mother is truly in labor—that is, her cervix is dilating.

If you are aware of these signs of labor, chances are very good that you will be able to correctly interpret what is going on. Sometimes, though, couples need the help of the caregiver to figure out if the mother is really in labor or not.

Signs and Symptoms	Comments
Possible Signs	
Vague nagging backache causing restlessness—a need to keep changing positions.	• Different from the fatigue-related backache that is common during pregnancy. • May be associated with early contractions.
Several soft bowel movements—sometimes accompanied by flu-like, "sick" feelings.	• When this sign accompanies others, it is probably associated with an increase in hormone-like substances in the bloodstream (prostaglandins). These substances soften and thin the cervix and stimulate bowel activity. By itself, however, this symptom may be due to a digestive upset.
Cramps, similar to menstrual cramps, that come and go; the discomfort may extend to the thighs.	• May be associated with prostaglandin action and early contractions. •May go away and return several times or progress steadily to positive signs.
Unusual burst of energy resulting in great activity (cleaning, organizing); this is termed the "nesting urge."	• Ensures that the mother will have strength and energy to handle labor (but she should try to curb exhausting activity).
Preliminary Signs	
Blood-tinged mucous discharge ("show" or mucous plug) released from the vagina; mother continues passing this discharge off and on throughout labor.	• Associated with thinning of the cervix. • May occur days before other signs or not until after progressing contractions have begun. • A discharge, often mistaken for show, may also appear within a day after a prenatal pelvic examination or sexual intercourse and is not a sign of labor. Show is pink or red; the discharge after a pelvic exam or sex tends to be brownish.
Bag of waters leaks, resulting in a trickle of fluid from the vagina, but no contractions occur. (See "If Her Bag of Waters Breaks Before Labor Begins," page 48.)	• Occurs before labor only about 10 to 13 percent of the time. • A signal to call the caregiver.

Signs and Symptoms	Comments
Continuing, nonprogressing contractions that do *not* become longer, stronger, and closer together over a period of time. These are prelabor, or Braxton-Hicks, contractions. (See "'False' Labor, or Prelabor," page 49.)	• Accomplishes softening and thinning of the cervix, preparing the cervix to begin dilating. • Should not be perceived as unproductive. • These are usually not painful, but they may be tiring or discouraging if they continue for many hours.

Positive Signs

Progressing contractions—that is, contractions that become longer, stronger, and closer together over time. These usually continue until it is time to push. Some women having second or subsequent babies, however, have periods of progressing contractions that come and go over a few days before they settle into a continuous pattern.	• A clear sign that the cervix is opening are 10 to 12 contractions that (1) consistently average 1 minute in length, (2) occur 5 or fewer minutes apart, and (3) feel painful or "very strong." • It is an even clearer sign if these contractions are combined with a "show" (blood-tinged discharge). • The mother cannot be distracted from these contractions. • She may feel these contractions in her abdomen or back, or both.
Spontaneous breaking of the bag of waters (rupture of the membranes) with a pop or gush of fluid followed by progressing contractions within hours. (See "If Her Bag of Waters Breaks Before Labor Begins," page 48.)	• Often associated with rapid labor. • The bag of waters usually breaks in late labor. Rupture of the membranes occurs before other signs of labor only about 10 percent of the time.

SIGNS OF LABOR

CAUTION: If the mother experiences noticeable contractions (every 15 minutes or less) for more than two hours, combined with *any* of the other Possible, Preliminary, or Positive signs of labor *more than three weeks before her due date*, she should tell her caregiver. She might be in *premature labor*, which can sometimes be stopped if it is caught early. If she is beyond 37 weeks of pregnancy, she should wait for the Positive Signs before calling her caregiver.

If Her Bag of Waters Breaks
Before Labor Begins

If the mother's membranes rupture (if water leaks or flows from her vagina) before labor begins, make the following observations to report to her caregiver:

1. *The amount* of fluid. Is it a trickle, a squirt when she changes position, or a gush?

2. The *color* of the fluid. Normally, the fluid is clear. If it is brownish or greenish, the baby may have emptied his bowels (passed meconium), which happens when a baby is stressed in the uterus. Such stress is caused by a temporary lack of oxygen.

3. The *odor* of the fluid. Normally, the fluid is practically odorless. If it has a foul smell, there may be an infection within the uterus, which could spread to the baby.

This information helps the caregiver plan what to do next—have the mother stay home, with some precautions, come into the office for an examination, or go to the hospital.

A concern with ruptured membranes is whether the mother is a carrier of Group B streptococcus. If so, she will be offered antibiotics to prevent an infection in the baby (see page 181).

Also, once the bag of waters has broken, the mother should take precautions to prevent bacteria from entering her uterus, increasing the chance of infection. She should put nothing in her vagina: She should not use tampons; she should not have intercourse; she should not check her cervix with her fingers. She *can* take a tub bath, which will not increase the chance of infection, but do be sure the tub is clean.

The caregiver and nurses should be very cautious about doing vaginal exams. Exams tend to push bacteria up into the uterus and increase the chances of infection. Vaginal exams are often done out of curiosity—simply to find out if the cervix has changed. With a broken bag of waters, it is safer to restrict vaginal exams to situations in which (a) a decision needs to be made about how to proceed (for example, whether to induce labor—start labor with medications—or allow the mother to walk, and so forth), *and* (b) the decision depends on how much the cervix has already changed or on other factors that can be determined only with a vaginal exam.

If these precautions are followed, the mother can probably safely wait for labor to begin spontaneously, and the caregiver probably won't think that it is necessary to induce labor. Most caregivers have a policy regarding their management of ruptured membranes (broken bag of waters); some want to induce labor within hours after the bag breaks, whereas others wait. It is wise to find out this policy ahead of time and try to change it if the mother is uncomfortable with it.

CAUTION: On very rare occasions, the baby's cord slips out of the uterus as the water escapes. This is called *prolapsed cord* and is a *true emergency*. See "Prolapsed Cord," page 213.

"False" Labor, or Prelabor

Frequently, women have contractions that seem quite strong and frequent, but when examined they are told they are in "false" labor, which means the cervix is not yet opening (dilating). The term *prelabor* is much more appropriate, because there is nothing "false" about these contractions, and they are accomplishing changes that allow "true" labor (that is, dilation) to occur. Prelabor contractions, also called Braxton-Hicks contractions, may occur frequently in late pregnancy. Besides being discouraged, many women in prelabor feel embarrassed or worried, and they may lose faith in their ability to recognize labor. The kind of labor support the mother receives under these circumstances is critical to her ability to cope with "true," progressing labor later on. Here is how you can help:

- It is most important to point out that "false" labor does not mean that what the mother is experiencing is not real. All it means is that her cervix has not yet begun to open. Refer to the contractions as "prelabor."
- Remind her that opening (dilation) of the cervix beyond about 2 centimeters is one of the *last* things to happen in labor. The fact that her cervix is not yet opening does *not* mean that she is not making progress.

- If the mother becomes discouraged with a prolonged period of little or no apparent progress, remind her of the six ways her body may be progressing (see "Labor Progresses in Six Ways" below).
- Ask the caregiver who examines the mother if the cervix has moved forward, if it has softened further, or if it has thinned more. Sometimes the caregiver is so focused on the opening of the cervix (dilation), he or she fails to mention these other important signs of progress.
- See "Prelabor," page 60, and "The Slow-to-Start Labor," page 135, for some strategies to help the mother cope with these early contractions.

You can be sure that if the mother has either of the Positive Signs of labor listed in the table on page 47, her cervix is opening. She cannot be in "false" labor if, over a period of time, her contractions have become longer *and* stronger *and* closer together. See "Timing Contractions," page 53.

Labor Progresses in Six Ways

A woman makes progress toward birth in the following ways. Note that significant dilation does not take place until step 4.

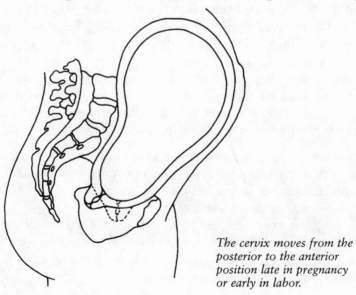

The cervix moves from the posterior to the anterior position late in pregnancy or early in labor.

The first three steps usually take place simultaneously and gradually over the last weeks of pregnancy.

1. *The cervix softens (ripens)*. While still thick, the cervix, through the action of hormones and prostaglandins, softens and becomes more pliable.

2. *The position of the cervix changes*. The cervix points toward the mother's back during most of pregnancy, then gradually moves forward. The position of the cervix is assessed by a vaginal exam and is described as posterior (pointing toward the back), midline, or anterior (pointing toward the front).

3. *The cervix thins and shortens (effaces)*. Usually about 1½ inches long, the cervix gradually shortens and becomes paper-thin. The amount of thinning (effacement) is measured in two ways:

- *Percentages*. Zero percent means no thinning or shortening has occurred; 50 percent means the cervix is about half its former thickness; 100 percent means it is paper-thin.
- *Centimeters of length*. Three to four centimeters long is the same as 0 percent effaced; 2 centimeters long is the same as 50 percent effaced; and less than 1 centimeter long means 80 to 90 percent effaced. Be sure not to confuse centimeters of cervical length with centimeters of cervical dilation!

4. *The cervix opens (dilates)*. The opening (dilation) of the cervix is also measured in centimeters. Dilation usually occurs with progressing contractions—after the cervix has undergone

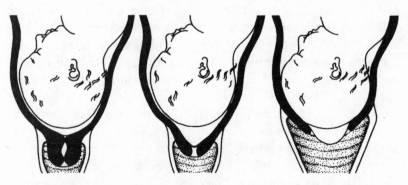

A cervix that has not effaced or dilated, and is 3 to 4 cm long

A cervix that is 75 percent effaced (about 1 cm long), and 1 cm dilated

A cervix that is 100 percent effaced (or paper-thin) and 4 cm dilated

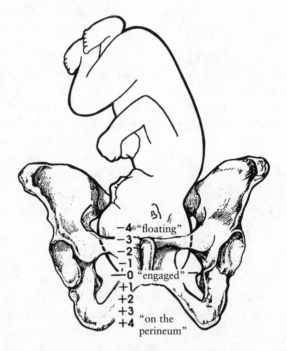

Station—a measure of the baby's descent.

the changes just described—but it is common for the cervix to dilate 1 to 3 centimeters before the woman has positive signs of labor. The cervix must open to approximately 10 centimeters (almost 4 inches) in diameter to allow the baby through.

5. *The baby's head rotates.* This rotation makes it easier for the baby to pass through the birth canal. (Sometimes the head must "mold" before it can rotate. This means that the head changes shape, becoming longer and thinner. Molding is normal, although some babies' heads look somewhat misshapen for a day or two following birth, after which time the head returns to a round shape.) The most favorable position for birth is usually the OA (occiput anterior) position. See page 44 for information on other positions.

6. *The baby descends.* The baby descends through the cervix, the pelvis, and the vagina to the outside. The descent is described in terms of "station," which (a) tells how far above or below the mother's mid-pelvis is the baby's head (or buttocks, in the case

of a breech presentation—see page 160 for more information about breech presentation); (b) is measured in centimeters; and (c) ranges from "minus 4" to "plus 4" ("0 station" means the baby's head is right at the mother's mid-pelvis). "Minus 1, 2, 3, or 4" means the head is that number of centimeters above the mid-pelvis. The greater the "plus" number, the closer the baby's head is to the outside and to being born.

Some descent takes place before labor begins, especially with first-time mothers. When the baby *drops*, it settles into the pelvis. Most descent, however, does not occur until late in labor.

Steps 4 to 6 (dilation beyond 2 to 3 centimeters, rotation, and descent) cannot take place until the first three steps are well underway. In other words, a cervix that is firm, thick, or posterior won't open. It simply is not ready. And a baby won't rotate and descend significantly until the cervix is open. For many women the first three steps take place imperceptibly and gradually in late pregnancy. For others they take place all at once, with hours or days of frequent and sometimes strong or even painful nonprogressing contractions, referred to as "prelabor," or Braxton-Hicks contractions.

Timing Contractions

In early labor, one of the important jobs of the birth partner is to time contractions. Since changes in the length, strength, and frequency of contractions are the all-important hallmarks of true, progressing labor, it is a good idea for you to (1) know how to time correctly and (2) keep a written record. Then, when you call the mother's caregiver, you will have accurate and concrete information to provide.

Time contractions in this way:

1. Use a watch or clock with a second hand.
2. Use a written form similar to the sample "Early Labor Record," page 54.
3. You do not need to time every contraction. Instead, time and record five or six contractions in a row and then stop for a while (a few minutes to a few hours). Skip a line on the form to separate the timing periods. Time and record another five or six

Date _____

Time Contraction Starts	Duration (seconds)	Interval (minutes from start of one to start of next)	Comments (contraction strength, foods eaten, breathing pattern, vaginal discharge, etc.)

contractions later, when the mother thinks they have changed or when she has had some of the other signs of labor.

4. Always note the time each contraction begins (specify A.M. or P.M.). Record this time in the column headed "Time Contraction Starts."

5. Time the length of each contraction (in seconds), and record this time in the column headed "Duration." Contractions usually range from 20 to 30 seconds long in pre- or early labor and 1½ to 2 minutes in late labor. Knowing when a contraction begins and ends is tricky. The best way is for the mother to signal when she feels the contraction begin and end. The mother can usually feel a contraction for longer, from the "inside," than can a nurse, who from the "outside" probably feels only the peak.

6. Figure out how frequently the contractions are coming by subtracting the time at the start of one contraction from the time at the start of the next. Record the number of minutes between contractions in the "Interval" column. (For example, if one contraction begins at 7:32 and the next one begins at 7:45, they are 13 minutes apart.) Do the same for each subsequent contraction.

7. In the "Comments" column, record anything else that may be significant: how strong the contractions seem now compared with earlier, the mother's appetite and what she has eaten, if she is using patterned breathing or other coping rituals (see page 105), if she has back pain or blood-tinged discharge, if fluid is leaking or gushing, how she is coping.

When you call her caregiver or the hospital's labor floor, be prepared to report the items on the "Early Labor Record." Have it near the phone. (Be sure you know whom to call. Some caregivers prefer that you call them directly; others want you to call the hospital.)

See page 66 for the discussion "When Do You Go to the Hospital or Settle In for a Home Birth?"

TIMING CONTRACTIONS

3

Moving Through the Stages of Labor

Labor and birth are among the most intense of all normal human experiences—physical, psychological, and mental. This is true not only for the woman, but also for those who love and care for her. Labor is unpredictable, empowering, and fulfilling, and it comes with a great prize at the end!

Childbirth has many similarities to a marathon or other physical-endurance event. Both include pain and psychological demands on the participant. Both become much more manageable when the participant has adequate preparation and the following inner and outer resources:

- Knowledge of what to expect.
- Prior planning with a knowledgeable guide.
- Physical health and fitness.
- Encouragement and support before and throughout the event.
- Confidence that muscle pain and fatigue are normal side effects of such effort.
- Fluids and adequate nourishment.

- The ability to pace oneself.
- The availability of expert medical assistance, in case it is needed.

It is true for both athletes and birthing women that if they develop complications, or begin to worry about the tough challenges ahead, or become preoccupied with their pain, or lose confidence, or become overwhelmed, they will have to adjust. The athlete may have to slow down or drop out; the laboring woman may have to change her plans and rely more on her caregiver to help her give birth in a safe and satisfying way.

The meaning of the event (the race or the labor) varies among endurance athletes and childbearing women alike. For some athletes, running a marathon means not only finishing, but also coming in at the front of the pack. For others, finishing is the goal and the reward. For some childbearing women, labor and birth represent not only having a baby, but also doing it without medical or surgical intervention. For others, having the baby is the goal and the reward.

The analogy between an endurance sporting event and childbirth breaks down, however, when we look further. One of the greatest differences is the matter of choice. Marathon runners do not have to run the race. They choose to do so. Healthy pregnant women, however, must go through labor and delivery (or another demanding and painful process—cesarean delivery) if they are to have children. The other enormous difference between the two events is their degree of predictability. The marathon runner knows when the event will take place and how long the course is, and can study and jog the course ahead of time. The course doesn't change and is the same for all participants.

The most predictable thing about birth is its total unpredictability. A pregnant woman does not know when it will begin, how long it will take, or how painful it will be, and she certainly does not know whether or how it might be similar or different from her mother's labors or the labors of other women. She cannot even be sure to have had a good night's sleep beforehand! And she certainly cannot predict what her postpartum course will be like.

This unpredictability of birth may be a source of frustration as you try to learn what to expect and how to help. Partners in my childbirth classes often ask me questions like these:

- Once the cervix has begun to ripen, how long does it usually take before labor starts?
- After contractions begin, how many hours before we should go to the hospital?
- How long is the pushing stage?
- When should I take time off from work?
- How bad is the pain?
- What do contractions feel like?

Birth partners want to know exactly what to prepare for, but it is simply not possible to answer these questions. Variations are inherent in childbirth, because each human being is unique.

This chapter will give you a broad idea of what you can expect from this mysterious process. You will learn of the wide range of normal possibilities, and how you can be truly helpful. The emotions experienced by laboring women constitute a large part of the discussion, along with the emotional responses that you as the birth partner may experience. Lastly, I will try to give you practical and useful suggestions to help you with the challenging task of providing the mother with emotional support as well as physical comfort.

The following medical terms describe what is happening during labor and how the mother is progressing:

- *Prelabor* describes the time before actual labor begins, when the mother is having nonprogressing contractions and her cervix isn't dilating. The contractions may come and go for a period of days.
- The *first stage* of labor is the *dilation stage*, during which the cervix dilates completely—to about 10 centimeters in diameter. The contractions progress; that is, they become longer, stronger, and/or closer together.
- The *second stage* is the *birthing stage*, during which the baby is born.
- The *third stage* is the *placental stage*, during which the placenta, or afterbirth, is born.

The dilation (first) and birthing (second) stages are further subdivided into three phases each. With every new phase, labor changes its rhythm, and the mother must make an emotional adjustment. This chapter describes each stage and phase, and includes suggestions about how you can help the mother cope. See the table "Normal Labor—in a Nutshell," pages 89–93, for a brief summary of this information.

Prelabor

What Is It? During prelabor, the mother has regular or off-and-on uterine contractions as the uterus begins "tuning up." The cervix softens, moves forward, and thins. Contractions may be regular and strong, and sometimes even fairly close together (every 6 to 8 minutes), for hours. However, they do not progress (by becoming longer, stronger, or closer together), and they may stop. The cervix is not yet dilating—the sign that she is truly in labor.

Prelabor is sometimes confusing to the mother, to her birth partner, and even to her caregiver. You may find it difficult to distinguish between this tuning up and the "real thing." Then, without warning, and perhaps without either of you recognizing it, prelabor contractions will become the "real thing": They will get longer, stronger, and/or closer together. The cervix will begin to dilate.

How Long Does It Last? Prelabor may last just a few hours, or come and go over several days.

How Will the Mother Feel? During prelabor, the mother may feel one or more of these emotions:

- *Confusion*, about whether she is in labor or not.
- *Excitement and anticipation*, as she realizes she will have the baby soon.
- *Fear or dread*, especially if she is not mentally prepared, if labor is earlier than she expected, or if her contractions are more painful than she expected.

If prelabor goes on for days, the mother may feel one or more of these emotions:

- *Frustration*, over not knowing what is happening and feeling tricked by the confusing signs.

- *Discouragement*, over the long wait.
- *Fatigue*, if she has missed sleep.
- *Doubt or anxiety*, about her body's ability to function properly, especially if the contractions are painful but not progressing (getting longer, stronger, and closer together).
- *Worry*, about being too tired to handle the progressing contractions when they begin.

What Does the Caregiver Do? Depending on your report, the caregiver may suggest that the mother wait at home, come in to the office for a progress check, or go straight to the hospital. In addition, the caregiver may do any of the following:

- Come to the home to check the mother if the birth is to take place there.
- Offer advice and encouragement to help her handle this frustrating phase.
- Suggest a warm bath or drugs for rest or to slow contractions if prelabor has been going on for a long time.
- Try to speed labor with drugs or by breaking the bag of waters (see "Induction or Augmentation of Labor," page 189).

How Might You Feel?

- Confusion, since you have no frame of reference against which to compare her present behavior or verbal expression of pain ("This seems easy" or "How much harder can this get?" or "I can't believe the nurse told us not to come in yet").
- Anxiety about packing the car and getting to the hospital in time.
- Frustration that prelabor seems to be taking so long or that the signs of labor are not clearer.
- Concern over whether you are helping her enough.
- Excitement that the big day is here (or near)!
- Eagerness to help the mother and see the baby.

How Can You Help? Help the mother with prelabor in these ways:

- Realize that a long prelabor is not a medical problem in itself. Therefore, it is mostly up to the two of you to handle it, perhaps with the help of a doula, friends, or family members.

- Recognize prelabor for what it is. Help the mother determine whether her contractions are progressing by timing them occasionally. (See "Timing Contractions," page 53; "Signs of Labor," page 44; and "'False' Labor, or Prelabor" page 49.)
- Check with the caregiver for advice and reassurance, and possibly to arrange for an examination.
- Encourage the mother to eat when she is hungry and drink when she is thirsty.
- Do projects or activities together. You might give her a massage, or the two of you might prepare food, go for walks, visit with friends, or read a book aloud to each other (one couple I know enjoyed reading a Harry Potter book as labor was starting).
- Consult "The Slow-to-Start Labor," page 137, for specific coping techniques if prelabor continues for a long time.

Dilation

What Is It? Dilation, or the opening of the cervix, occurs in the first stage of labor. Dilation begins when the prelabor contractions change their pattern and start getting longer, stronger, and/or closer together. The first stage ends when the cervix has dilated completely (to approximately 10 centimeters). Dilation can proceed very quickly or rather slowly. It has distinct phases: the latent phase (early labor); the active phase (active labor); and the transition phase (transition).

The line between prelabor and the dilation stage is rarely clear, so don't expect that you or the mother will know the moment her cervix begins to open.

In a typical labor, the contractions gradually and steadily increase in intensity and duration and come closer together. Early contractions may last 30 to 40 seconds and come every 15 to 20 minutes. Although there are exceptions, these early contractions are usually painless. But by the time the cervix has opened to 8 or 9 centimeters, the contractions may last 90 seconds, feel very intense (almost surely very painful), and come every 2 to 4 minutes. The pain of contractions usually reaches its maximum by 7 or 8 centimeters dilation (second-stage contractions, however, are very painful in another way).

Occasionally, labor does not follow this predictable pattern. Sometimes the early contractions are very painful and progress very quickly. If that is the case, there will be no time for you to use the following information. Skip to "The Very Rapid Labor," page 141, for help with this special situation.

How Long Does It Last? The dilation stage lasts from two to twenty-four hours. However, for first-time mothers it is rare for the dilation stage to last less than four hours.

You cannot know in advance how long dilation will take. Therefore, prepare yourselves for the whole range of possibilities: be able to handle the short, intense labor or to pace yourselves through the extra-long one. (See "The Very Rapid Labor," page 141; "The Slow-to-Start Labor," page 137; and "Slow Progress in Labor," page 210.)

When Should You Call the Caregiver or the Labor and Delivery Floor? Call under any of the following circumstances:

- If the mother has possible premature labor (see "Signs of Labor," page 45).
- If she has leaking or a gush of fluid (see "If Her Bag of Waters Breaks Before Labor Begins," page 48).
- When the mother's contractions are clearly becoming longer, stronger, and closer together (see "Signs of Labor," page 45, and "Timing Contractions," page 53).
- Whenever you or the mother has questions or concerns.
- If the mother has had a child before, she should call the caregiver or hospital whenever she thinks or knows she's in labor. A second (or later) labor is usually faster than a first one.

Early Labor

What Is It? The early labor phase (or early labor) is a subdivision of the dilation stage, and it begins when dilation begins. It lasts until the cervix is dilated to 4 or 5 centimeters. Medical professionals call this the *latent phase* of the first stage.

The big difference between prelabor and early labor is that during early labor the cervix begins to gradually open. Progressing contractions are the mother's best sign that early labor has begun. The caregiver uses vaginal exams as necessary to determine changes in the cervix during this phase.

How Long Does It Last? Typically, early labor takes from two-thirds to three-quarters of the total time of the dilation stage. In other words, it could take from a few hours to twenty hours or so for a woman to reach 4 centimeters of dilation. The length of early labor depends largely on the state of the cervix and on the position and station of the baby within the pelvis at the time labor begins. Chances for more rapid progress are increased if the following conditions exist:

- The cervix is very soft and thin.
- The baby is in the occiput anterior (OA) position, with his head down, his chin on his chest, and the back of his head toward the mother's front (see page 44).
- The baby is low in the mother's pelvis (see page 52).

These favorable conditions increase the likelihood of an average or shorter-than-average early labor. Under any other conditions, early labor is likely to take longer. Labor is not a race against time, however. A normal early labor can last from a few hours to many hours.

How Will the Mother Feel? The mother's response to early labor is not all that different from her response to prelabor. She is still uncertain. She still wants and looks for the positive signs of labor.

Getting into labor emotionally takes time. How the mother adjusts will depend on the circumstances—whether labor is early, on time, or late, and whether early contractions are hard and fast or vague and slow.

Reactions to labor range from relief, elation, or excitement to denial, disbelief, or panic. As labor settles into a rhythmic pattern, the mother settles down emotionally, pacing herself and finding routines for handling each contraction.

Sometimes, in the excitement of early labor, the mother

rushes the labor along in her mind. She may overreact or become preoccupied with every contraction. This results partly from her desire for labor to go quickly and partly from not knowing what level of intensity to expect. Without this frame of reference she may easily become convinced that her labor is progressing more rapidly than it really is.

When a woman rushes her labor mentally, she may go to the hospital too early, start using breathing techniques and other labor-coping measures before they are really needed, and, along with her partner, speculate that her cervix is dilated much more than it really is. Then, when she has a vaginal exam, she becomes discouraged to find that she's not nearly as advanced in labor as she thought she was.

How can you tell if the mother is (1) overreacting to early labor or (2) having a particularly difficult or rapid labor? Without vaginal exams, you cannot really know whether labor is progressing quickly or not. The best you can do is make an educated guess. Refer to "Signs of Labor" (page 45), time the contractions, and see if the mother can be distracted. Try a walk outside, or phone or visit with friends or relatives. If labor seems to "slow down" or become easier when the mother is distracted, she may have overreacted. Keep up the distractions (see "How You Can Help," page 90, for other ideas for handling an overreaction to early labor). Above all, try not to overreact yourself.

If labor does not slow down when you try to distract her, the mother is not overreacting. Stop trying to distract her, and, instead, encourage her to focus on her contractions. Help her to cope with this intense early labor.

What Does the Caregiver or Labor and Delivery Staff Do?
During early labor, the caregiver or hospital staff can help in the following ways:

- By giving advice over the telephone. When you call, be prepared to provide the information recorded on the Early Labor Record (page 54).
- By helping the mother decide when to go to the hospital or, if she is having a home birth, when to settle in at home for the labor.

- By doing a vaginal exam to give you both an idea of how the labor is progressing.

When Do You Go to the Hospital or Settle In for a Home Birth?
Under most circumstances, the first-time mother should go to the hospital or, if the birth will be at home, settle in there, when she has had *10 to 12* consecutive contractions that

- Last at least 1 minute.
- Average 5 or fewer minutes apart.
- Are strong enough that she *must* use a breathing, relaxation, or attention-focusing ritual (page 98).
- Are strong enough that she cannot be distracted from them.

It will take you and the mother about an hour to time these contractions and determine whether they fit this pattern.

Sometimes there are special reasons for the mother to go to the hospital earlier. For example:

- The mother lives a long distance from the hospital.
- She has medical problems that require early admission. Her caregiver should advise her if these problems exist.
- The mother has had a child before and recognizes that she is in labor. A woman's second (or later) labor usually goes faster than her first one did.
- She simply feels more secure in the hospital.

Because early labor can take so long, it is often a good idea to spend the time relaxing together by yourselves or with friends until the mother's contractions fit the pattern described here. It is usually best not to arrive at the hospital (or call the caregiver to the home) too early because

- The mother may feel "performance anxiety"—pressure to start producing some good contractions. Feeling watched by her caregiver or nurse, who seems to be waiting for something to happen, she may feel embarrassed that labor is so slow.
- The mother may become preoccupied with the contractions and the apparent lack of progress, making labor seem longer or more difficult than it is.
- The mother may become bored, anxious, or discouraged; she may become more likely to consider inappropriate medical interventions to speed up this normally slow part of labor.

Sometimes the caregiver will suggest that the mother leave the hospital and come back later. For a home birth, everyone except you may have to leave for a while. Although discouraging, these measures allow the labor to settle into its own pattern and take pressure off the mother.

How Might You Feel? You may have many of the feelings described for prelabor, plus

- Hope and elation, now that you notice the contractions progressing.
- Concern, especially if the mother is tired, discouraged, or having trouble dealing with the pain.
- Eagerness to get word from "the experts" that this is labor, that it is time to go to the hospital or for the midwife and others to arrive for a home birth.

How Can You Help? Your role now is not very different from the role you played during prelabor. You can help in these ways:

- Remain close by.
- Supply the mother with food and drink.
- Time five or six contractions, as described on page 53, when the pattern seems to change.
- Help the mother pass the time with pleasant and distracting activities. Refer to the activities suggested for "The Slow-to-Start Labor," page 137.
- Talk with the mother if you feel you should leave for work, errands, or other activities. Your decision should be based on her feelings and the following considerations:

    Are you always accessible by phone? Some birth partners carry cell phones or rent pagers (see "Paging Systems" in the Yellow Pages) for a few weeks before the due date so they will always be within reach.

    How far would you have to travel to reach the mother? How long would it take you?

    Is there someone else available (a friend, a relative, a neighbor) to help out if the mother needs someone right away?

    What are the pressures on you—from work, school, or other responsibilities? Will a few more hours really let you clear up pressing obligations?

If you feel you should leave, and the mother agrees, be sure someone else sits in for you until you are free. This should be a last resort.

Sooner or later, the labor pattern will intensify and the mother will become preoccupied with the contractions. She will no longer be able to walk or talk through them without pausing, and it will no longer be appropriate to distract her. Instead, you now need to do the following:

- Give the mother your undivided attention throughout every contraction. Stop what you are doing and stop talking so you can focus on her. Do not ask her questions during contractions.
- Watch her during the contractions and help her to relax her entire body during each one (see "Relaxation," page 102).
- Suggest that she begin using patterned breathing (see page 105).
- Give her encouragement during the contractions ("That's good. . . . Just like that"), and helpful comments when the contraction is over ("You relaxed very well that time," or "I noticed you tensed your shoulders with that contraction; with the next one, try to keep your shoulders relaxed").
- Help her decide when to call her caregiver.

Early labor eventually settles into a clear pattern of contractions, resulting in the more rapid dilation of the cervix—the active labor phase.

Active Labor

What Is It? The active phase of labor (or active labor) begins when the cervix has dilated to 4 or 5 centimeters and lasts until it reaches about 8 centimeters. During active labor the rhythm and pace of labor change, and the mother's cervix opens more steadily and more rapidly than it did during early labor. The cervix is now so thin and soft that it offers much less resistance to dilation.

During active labor, contractions tend to be clear-cut, consistently lasting at least a full minute and averaging 3 to 5 minutes apart. They are usually very intense, and most women describe them as painful.

It is important to recognize active labor and its positive meanings. It means labor is progressing well. It means that the mother will benefit from a quiet room, as free as possible from unnecessary disturbance. She will also benefit from the freedom to move around, in and out of bed. This is when women become more instinctual, more focused, less verbal. The mother may begin to moan and sway, to want to be held or stroked, or, conversely, not touched at all.

How Long Does It Last? Normally, active labor is shorter than early labor. For first-time mothers, active labor usually ranges from two to six hours. It is usually much faster for mothers who have had babies before—from 20 minutes to three hours.

What Does the Mother Feel? The mother must make an emotional adjustment to the changing rhythm of labor, for the following reasons:

- Labor has already continued for a relatively long time; prelabor and early labor may have been going on for hours or even for days.
- Then, when she is feeling that labor is very long, it also becomes more painful as the contractions pick up in strength and frequency.
- The mother may not yet realize why the contractions are increasing. Until some time has passed and she has made more progress, she may not be aware that her labor is speeding up.

The mother may respond to the changing rhythm of labor in the following ways:

- She may feel tired and discouraged as she realizes that the tough part is just beginning. She may lose confidence in her ability to cope with these more frequent, intense contractions.
- Her sense of humor fades. Your funniest jokes don't amuse her.
- Extraneous conversation becomes annoying. She may feel very alone if you and others do not recognize this change and continue trying to distract her, or, worse yet, ignore her.
- She becomes serious and focused on herself and her contractions. About all she can do is try to relax, breathe, and perhaps moan during her contractions. When a contraction

ends, most of her conversation may be centered on reviewing it with you and talking about what to do for the next one.

- She may become quiet; the room becomes quiet.
- For many women, the active labor phase is their "moment of truth." Suddenly it sinks in that this labor is real; there is no way out except to keep going and have the baby. Realizing this may frighten or depress her at first, but with help from you she can accept and yield to the labor, and work with it instead of trying to control it.
- As she realizes that she is not in control, she may fight against losing control, or feel panicky as she realizes she is caught up in this relentless process. She may weep and say it is too hard, that she cannot go on, or that she wants pain medications.
- With good support and freedom from disturbance, she will get past the crisis, release her need to control, and let her body take over. Her mood will settle in to acceptance, and she will find her own "rituals" (see chapter 4) for handling the contractions.

What Does the Caregiver Do? Unless there is a problem, the doctor is seldom at the bedside during active labor, but is available nearby or by telephone. A nurse provides most of the bedside care, following the doctor's orders. If the caregiver is a midwife, she usually provides care herself; otherwise, a nurse carries out the midwife's orders. During active labor, the midwife or nurse remains close by and becomes more actively involved. Now that progress is faster and the contractions are more intense, closer surveillance is needed. The nurse or the midwife frequently checks

- The mother's blood pressure, pulse, and temperature.
- Her fluid intake and urine output.
- The amount of dilation of her cervix.
- The fetal heart rate.
- The quality, intensity, and frequency of the contractions.
- Other signs.

Routines vary depending on the management style of the caregiver. Some caregivers rely heavily on interventions and medical technology. For example, they might break the bag of waters, keep the mother in bed, give intravenous (IV) fluids, use electronic monitors to check the fetus and the contractions, and give the mother medications to relieve pain. Other caregivers rely on simpler methods. They might encourage the mother to drink liquids and move around, listen to the fetal heartbeat with a stethoscope or a hand-held ultrasound device, and suggest comfort measures (page 95) to relieve pain. See the introduction to part 3, and chapter 6, for information about commonly used tests and procedures, as well as for questions to ask and alternatives to consider.

The nurse or the caregiver also offers advice and reassurance. Having someone there with expertise and experience—someone you both trust—can be immensely reassuring. Don't hesitate to ask for help or advice if you feel uncertain about the labor or about how you can help the mother.

How Might You Feel? Active labor may be hard for you in several ways:

- Seeing the mother in pain, or weeping, or asking you to help her may make you feel ineffective, helpless, worried, or even a little guilty that she has to go through so much.
- If you do not recognize that her progress is probably speeding up, you may worry about how long the labor is taking, especially since it is so intense.
- You may feel anxious to relieve her pain and seek an anesthesiologist to give her an epidural.
- If you recognize that she is making good progress, you may feel encouraged and confident that she can do it and that you can help her.

How Can You Help? Your role during active labor is very important. How you respond to the mother's needs determines to a large extent how well she copes and how satisfied with her labor experience she will feel later. Here are some guidelines for helping the mother during this phase.

- *Be sure the staff is aware of her Birth Plan,* especially with her preferences regarding pain medications and other interventions.

- *Follow the mother's lead.* Take your cues from her; match her mood. When she becomes serious or quiet, you should become serious or quiet. Don't try to cheer her up or jolly her out of this mood.

  Do not continue trying to distract her. The labor takes almost all her attention, and she needs you with her both physically and emotionally.

- *Acknowledge her feelings* if she says, "I can't do this," with a comment such as "This is rough. Let me help you more. Keep your rhythm."

- *Give the mother your undivided attention* throughout every contraction, even if her eyes are closed and she seems not to need it. Do not chat with others in the room, and discourage others from engaging in nonessential conversation. Such talk could make the mother feel very alone and ignored, even if she is coping well. Help her to remain relaxed and use patterned breathing through each contraction (see "Relaxation," page 102, and "Rhythmic Breathing and Moaning Patterns," page 105).

- *Support her "ritual."* A *ritual*, in labor, is a series of comforting rhythmic actions, repeated during every contraction. Some rituals such as breathing, relaxation, and attention-focusing techniques are learned in advance, and are especially helpful in early labor.

  During contractions, you should always be looking for either stillness and relaxation or rhythmic ritual as signs that she is coping well. If she tenses, grimaces, writhes, clutches, or cries out, and there is no rhythm in her actions, she needs help. She needs you to help her maintain her rhythm as she moans, moves, or taps, by making eye contact or by rhythmically talking, stroking, or swaying along with her (see "The Three *R*s," page 97).

  You also might suggest a bath or shower, a new position, a walk, or counter-pressure to ease her pain (see chapter 4).

Other rituals are discovered on the spot during labor. The basic ritual for handling contractions can include any of the many comfort measures described on pages 95 to 129 that appeal to the mother. Try to include as part of the ritual reminders to sip fluid after each contraction or two and empty her bladder every hour or two.

Don't be surprised when unexpected and unplanned personal touches—for example, speaking or moaning in a certain tone of voice, repeating particular words or phrases, feeling your touch (in a certain way in a certain spot), close eye contact, a series of movements—become vital parts of the mother's labor ritual. This is what usually happens. The mother's adaptation of a ritual to suit her own way of laboring is a very good sign. (See page 98 for more on rituals and examples of some that others have created.)

Stick with the same ritual for as long as it helps. Don't be afraid to try something new if the mother is not responding well. She will let you know if she wants to go back to the previous ritual.

Transition

What Is It? The transition phase is a turning point in labor; it is the period of transition from the dilation to the birthing stage. Professionals call this the transition from the first to the second stage because the mother's body seems to be partly in the dilation (first) stage and partly in the birthing (second) stage.

During the transition phase the cervix dilates the last 2 centimeters or so (from about 8 centimeters to about 10) to complete the dilation (first) stage of labor. At this time, the baby begins to descend—the head moves from the uterus through the cervix and down into the vagina—to begin the birthing (second) stage of labor. Contractions have reached their maximum intensity, last 1½ to 2 minutes, and occur very close together.

Sometimes a "lip" of cervix remains. A "lip" occurs when a part of the cervix remains thick after most of the cervix has completely dilated. The presence of a lip seems to delay the last bit of dilation. It may take several contractions before the cervix eases back to let the baby's head through.

The uterus may begin its expulsive efforts even before the cervix is completely dilated. We call this the "urge to push." It makes the mother catch her breath, grunt, or hold her breath and strain; this is what is meant by the terms "pushing" and "bearing down." The urge to push is an involuntary reflex; she does not make it happen and cannot prevent it from happening. Yet if the cervix is not completely dilated, it may be better if she tries to bear down very slightly—just enough to satisfy her urge. I call this "grunt-pushing." She may be asked to do this by the nurse or caregiver. Pushing very hard before the cervix is dilated could cause the cervix to swell and the labor to slow. (See "Avoiding Forceful Pushing," page 109.)

How Long Does It Last? The transition usually takes from five to twenty-five contractions; it lasts from fifteen minutes to an hour and fifteen minutes. If a lip of cervix remains, the transition phase is likely to take longer.

What Does the Mother Feel? Transition may be the most difficult part of labor for the mother. Even though the contractions are no more intense, their frequency combined with the sensations of the baby's head moving down may cause the mother's legs, or even her whole body, to tremble. She may feel nauseated and may vomit; vomiting usually brings relief. She may feel cramps in her thighs or pressure in her pelvis. She may feel she needs to pass a bowel movement. She may feel very hot, then cold. She may weep or cry out, feeling that she cannot handle any more, that labor will never end. She may feel overwhelmed, and react angrily, saying, "Don't touch me! My skin hurts!" or "I can't go on!" or "Stop doing that!" Or she may withdraw into herself, dozing between contractions and moaning, groaning, or whimpering during them, all the while relaxing her body quite well. Transition affects different women differently, but all are relieved when this phase is over.

What Does the Caregiver Do? During the transition phase, a nurse or a midwife is in constant attendance. The doctor is not necessarily with the mother, although when informed that the mother is approaching delivery, the doctor soon comes.

The nurse or the midwife does the following:

- Checks the cervix if she needs to confirm the mother's progress in labor.
- Asks the mother not to push or to push only gently if the cervix is not fully opened.

- Offers reassurance that the mother is all right and that labor is moving rapidly.
- Helps you in your role as birth partner and reassures you that the mother is all right and behaving normally.
- Begins preparations for the birth.

If the birth will take place in the same room where the mother is laboring, the nurse or the midwife brings in the equipment necessary for the delivery and for the immediate care of the baby. If the birth is to take place in a separate delivery room, the staff prepares to take the mother there, bed and all. Be sure to go along!

This is an exciting moment, when everyone begins preparing for the infant. Finally, even the staff is acting as if a baby is really coming!

How Might You Feel? You may feel as if you are caught up in a flurry of activity and intense feelings.

- You may be tired, especially if the labor has gone through the night.
- You may have been wondering if she would ever reach complete dilation and feel surprised as she nears that goal.
- You may feel helpless in the face of her pain, wishing you could do something to erase it.
- You may feel frustrated or hurt, if she seems to find fault with everything you try to do to help.
- You may want to take a break, but she pleads, "Don't leave! I need you!"
- You may worry, wondering if such a demanding labor is normal.

How Can You Help? Your role during transition is all important. You can truly take some of the mother's burden if you know what to do:

- Help her maintain a rhythmic ritual (see page 98).
- Stay calm. Your touch should be firm and confident. Your voice should remain calm and encouraging.
- Stay close to the mother with your face near hers.

- If she is panicky and scared, go into your "Take-Charge Routine" (page 134).
- Remind her that this difficult phase is short, that she is almost in the birthing stage, and that the contractions are as painful as they will get. Help her get through one contraction at a time.
- Remind yourself that it is *normal* for the transition phase to be difficult, that the mother's mood will improve when her cervix is fully dilated, and that if you are to reassure her you must not worry about her. Her behavior is not abnormal; her pain is not more than one should expect at this time. The rest of labor will not be this intense.
- What about pain medications? If the mother has planned to use pain medications during labor, she can take them now (use the "Pain Medications Preference Scale," pages 249 to 251, to guide your decisions). If she has wanted to avoid pain medications, then do not mention them. Instead, help her get through this phase without them, as tough as it may be.
- Be sure the nurse or caregiver knows if the mother has an urge to push (see page 73). The caregiver will check the mother's progress to determine if pushing is appropriate.
- If the caregiver says the mother isn't ready to push yet, help her to avoid pushing, or to push with little grunts (see "Breathing Patterns for Pushing," page 109).
- Try not to take it personally if the mother criticizes you. She is expressing that labor is so difficult right now that nothing helps. You are the safest person for her to lash out at. Later, she will probably apologize.

Descent and Birth

What Is It? The birthing stage, or stage of descent, begins when the cervix is fully dilated and ends with the birth of the baby. Medical professionals call it the *second stage.*

During the birthing stage the mother works very hard: She bears down—actively pushes—by holding her breath and straining or breathing out forcefully with the urge to push that comes several times in every contraction. In this way she works with her uterus to press the baby down and out. The birthing stage

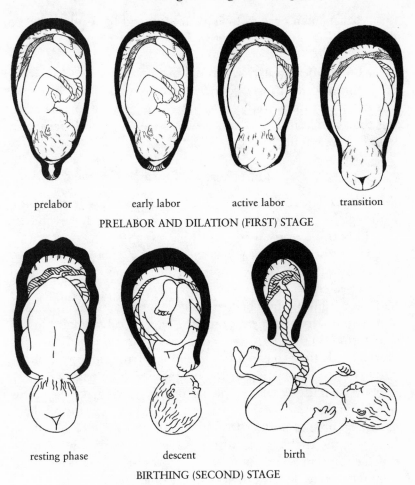

prelabor   early labor   active labor   transition

PRELABOR AND DILATION (FIRST) STAGE

resting phase   descent   birth

BIRTHING (SECOND) STAGE

The baby rotates and descends as the cervix opens.

has three distinct phases: the resting, the descent, and the crowning and birth phases (see the illustrations above). Each phase is characterized by different physical developments, and each requires that the mother make an emotional adjustment.

The management of the birthing (second) stage varies among caregivers. Some want to speed the baby's descent with drugs and instruments, whereas others feel it is better to let the labor unfold at its own pace as long as mother and baby appear to be doing well.

How Long Does It Last? A normal birthing stage may last from 15 minutes (three to five contractions) to three hours or more. For most first-time mothers, the birthing stage is completed in less than two hours; for women who have given birth before, in less than one hour.

The Resting Phase

What Is It? The resting phase is an apparent pause in the labor. Although not all women experience it, you and the mother should both be ready for it.

The resting phase is a "catch-up break" for the uterus; it comes after the cervix is completely dilated and the baby's head has passed through the cervix into the birth canal. The uterus had been tightly stretched around the baby before the head slipped out. Now, suddenly, only the baby's body remains inside the uterus and the uterus fits more loosely around the baby. The uterus needs time to catch up, to tighten around the rest of the baby. See the illustration of the resting phase on page 77.

Now the muscle fibers in the uterus shorten to make the uterus smaller, without noticeable contractions and without the mother's having an urge to push. The mother also gets a rest break. Sheila Kitzinger, the well-known British teacher and author, has termed this the "rest and be thankful phase." After the tumult of transition, the resting phases provides a welcome break.

How Long Does It Last? The resting phase usually lasts up to 30 minutes. If it lasts longer than that, most caregivers urge the mother to change position or to push (bear down) in an effort to speed labor along and bring on stronger contractions. They don't want labor to slow down for very long at this point.

What Does the Mother Feel? The start of the birthing stage is always a milestone. The mother will probably welcome this rest, especially after the tumult of transition. She gets "a new lease on life," a second wind. If she was confused, her head is now clear. If she was discouraged, she is now optimistic. If she was withdrawn, she is now outgoing and aware of her surroundings. Sometimes a woman feels anxious if the resting phase seems to go on for too long or if the staff is imploring her to push before she feels an urge to do so. She may also feel inadequate or apologetic if everyone is commanding her to push, making her feel as if she is not doing well enough. In fact, no one should be expecting her to push if she feels no urge. She should be allowed to rest.

Even women who do not experience a period of rest improve in mood at the beginning of the birthing stage.

What Does the Caregiver Do? During the resting phase

- The midwife or nurse remains close by, offering encouragement, praise, and positive suggestions.
- The nurse will probably call the doctor to come soon. If the mother has had a child before, the doctor will try to arrive soon after she begins pushing. If it is her first child, the doctor probably will not rush.
- The midwife or nurse may become more directive at this time, telling the mother what positions to try, or how or when to push.
- The midwife or nurse listens frequently to the baby's heartbeat and continues assessing the mother's welfare.
- The midwife or nurse may do a vaginal exam to assess the progress of the baby's descent.

How Might You Feel?

- The lifting of the mother's mood as she passes into the birthing stage is exciting. You will probably be relieved that she seems more like her usual self. (One woman looked up at her husband during this phase and asked, "Did you feed the cats?" Only 10 minutes before she had been moaning and tensing during contractions.)
- You may be baffled at the apparent stopping of her labor. Do not worry. The pause is temporary and will give the mother a second wind.
- You may feel overwhelmed at the realization that you are about to witness a miracle—the birth of this beloved baby.

How Can You Help? The birthing stage is an exciting time. But even though you have your own powerful emotional reaction to the birth, you are still the mother's major source of support, so you must remain calm and continue to encourage and assist her. Here are some guidelines:

- Be patient during the resting phase. Don't try to rush the mother through it or make her push too soon.
- If the nurse or caregiver wants the mother to push without a contraction or without the urge, ask if she can wait until she feels the urge to push.
- Match her mood. As she leaves the emotions of transition behind, you should do the same.
- Review with the mother and her caregiver what will be happening from now on, as the labor picks up again.
- If you are confused, ask the midwife or nurse what is going on.

The Descent Phase

What Is It? During the descent phase the uterus resumes contracting strongly, and the mother usually feels a strong urge to push. The baby descends through the birth canal to the point where the top of the head is clearly visible at the vaginal outlet. The mother alternately pushes and breathes lightly during contractions and rests between contractions.

By pushing, we mean that she holds her breath and strains for 5 to 6 seconds at a time. The push may be voluntary, meaning that she does it when she wants (or is told) to do it. Involuntary or spontaneous pushing occurs with the reflexive urge to push, which can be very powerful. One woman described it as "a vomit in reverse," meaning that she could feel it coming and could not resist it. Instead of everything coming up, all the force went down, pressing the baby out.

The baby's descent is usually intermittent; he moves down when the mother bears down during her urges to push, and slips back during the pauses between the mother's bearing-down efforts. You will find yourself totally engrossed in the moment. You almost hate to see the baby slip back each time because you're so anxious to see him born. You must remember that progress is being made, and this gradual stretching is easier on both baby and mother than constant pressure on the baby's head and continuous stretching of the vagina.

The mother may change positions during the descent phase. The best positions are semisitting, lying on one side, resting on hands and knees, and squatting. Supported squatting, "the dangle," and sitting on the toilet are also useful at times. See "Positions and Movements for Labor and Birth," page 112, which explains the benefits of each of these positions.

How Long Does It Last? The descent phase usually takes up most of the total time of the birthing stage—from a few minutes to three hours or so.

What Does the Mother Feel? The mother finds strength and determination during the descent phase, even after a long labor. The imminence of the birth heartens her, and she is receptive to suggestions and to praise. She may have other feelings as well:

- Early in the descent phase, especially, she may feel uncertain about what to do and how to do it. She may ask how she is doing, needing reassurance that her sensations are normal, that she is all right. She will do better after a few contractions.
- She may feel afraid to let go. This is the most difficult thing to do at this time—to let the baby come out. The sensations of descent and of the large solid head stretching the birth canal are gratifying and yet alarming and painful. It is scary to let the baby come *because it hurts*. She may instinctively resist the passage of the baby by tensing her pelvic floor against the baby's downward movement. If the mother did perineal massage during pregnancy, she will now find it easier to relax appropriately. (Prenatal perineal massage is a rehearsal for the sensations of the birthing stage, and it gives the mother a chance to practice relaxing while her vagina is being stretched. See "Prenatal Perineal Massage," page 21.)
- If the baby's descent is extremely rapid, the mother may feel shocked and frightened by the intensity of sensation and by her total lack of control over her body.
- If the descent is very slow, she will become discouraged. This may be the most demanding work of her entire life, and she needs to feel she is making progress.

What Does the Caregiver Do? During the descent phase

- The nurse or midwife continues as before, encouraging the mother's efforts and reassuring her.
- The doctor usually arrives during this phase, perhaps to your great relief.
- The doctor or midwife performs occasional vaginal exams to confirm the baby's progress. The nurse, midwife, or doctor checks the baby's heart rate and the mother's vital signs periodically.
- When the birth is imminent, the doctor or midwife scrubs and dons surgical gloves, special hospital clothing, and a mask.
- The nurse, doctor, or midwife may place drapes beneath the mother, may cleanse the mother's vaginal area, and may massage or place hot compresses on the perineum.
- The doctor or midwife uses his or her hands to control the emergence of the baby's head.

How Might You Feel?

- You recover from your fatigue and are ready to do whatever you are asked to do.
- You may feel divided between wanting to support the mother, remaining at her head, and wanting to watch the birth (or even catch the baby, with the help of the midwife or doctor).
- You may find yourself holding your breath right along with her!
- You may find yourself in an awkward position as you support her upper body or her leg. Your arms or back may tire. (This is one reason to try to improve your physical fitness before the birth; see page 21.)
- The initial excitement may fade to discouragement if progress seems too slow.

How Can You Help? With so many people around during the descent phase, you may feel less vital to the mother than you felt earlier. It is true that she now receives much of her direction and praise from others. This may be a relief to you because it allows you to become absorbed in your own experience of the birth. You are, however, still the mother's birth partner—the one who has seen her through all this—and she still may rely on you despite all of the attention from others. Here are some suggestions:

- Stay close to the mother, where she can see, feel, and hear you. You may support her from behind or by her side.
- Compliment her—tell her how well she is doing—with every contraction.
- Stay calm. Try to maintain a steady and reassuring tone of voice and a confident, firm touch (don't rub her or squeeze her too hard in your excitement); continue to encourage her.
- Do not keep telling her to push harder; you would only make her feel inadequate. Instead, encourage her: "That's the way! Come on, Baby."
- If she is not relaxing her perineum, remind her to "let go," "open up," or "let the baby out." Use whatever suggestions will help her release the tension in her perineum. Remind her to relax as she did during perineal massage (page 21) and during the "bulging" exercise (page 20). Request warm compresses to place on her perineum.
- Remind the mother that the baby is almost here! Sometimes, believe it or not, the mother almost forgets she is doing all this for her baby.
- If progress is slow, suggest that she try a different position. See "Positions and Movements for Labor and Birth," page 112, which explains the benefits of each of these positions. Be ready to support her in these positions.
- Remember that during a few contractions after the baby's head becomes visible at the vaginal opening, it may appear abnormal—wrinkled and spongy. Pressure on the head by the vaginal wall causes the skin of the scalp to be squeezed up to the top of the head (one birth partner thought it was a brain without a scalp!) until the head moves down more. Then it looks more as you would expect—hard and smooth.
- If the descent phase seems slow, try not to show your discouragement.

Few people are prepared for the power of the moment: the mother's superhuman effort; the sounds she makes; the baby bulging the vagina, peeking its wet and wrinkled scalp out, only to retreat yet again; the charged atmosphere of the room as everyone anticipates the birth. It is impossible to describe the awe, excitement, and tension you will feel as you await the moment of birth. However, don't forget that the mother still needs your support and attention.

The Crowning and Birth Phase

What Is It? The crowning and birth phase is when the baby is actually born. It is the transition from the birthing to the placental stage. It begins when the baby's head crowns—that is, when it remains visible at the vaginal opening even between contractions, no longer sneaking back between the mother's bearing-down efforts. This phase ends when the baby is born.

During the crowning and birth phase the mother's vagina and perineum are stretched more than at any other time, and they are more likely to sustain damage at this time than during any other phase. Protecting the perineum now becomes a major focus of the caregiver's management.

Until now, the baby's head has appeared wrinkled and spongy. Once the head crowns, the skin evens out over the scalp. The head seems to lurch forward a few times, and then it emerges—top of the head, brow and ears, then the face. The head rotates to one side, one shoulder appears, and the rest of the baby slides out with a gush of water.

At first the baby may appear blue and lifeless, but within seconds he begins breathing, usually with a gurgle, then a lusty cry. Immediately, the baby begins to turn more pink, and very soon he will be a healthy pink or ruddy color.

How Long Does It Last? The crowning and birth phase takes only a few contractions.

What Does the Mother Feel? The mother's body gives mixed messages during the crowning and birth phase: On the one hand, she knows the baby is almost here, and she is anxious to push hard to get him out quickly. On the other hand, she feels the stretching and burning (the "rim of fire") that signal her to stop pushing. To prevent the vagina or perineum from tearing, she should heed the message to stop pushing and ease the baby out, *not* push hard.

Although the crowning and birth are exciting for everyone else, this phase may be acutely painful for the mother, who has to devote all of her attention to getting the baby out. By the time the head is about to slip out, the pain has disappeared for some (but not all) women. The stretching of the vaginal outlet causes a temporary absence of the burning sensation. The mother may become alert, calm, and totally engrossed in greeting her baby—although this is less likely in a rapid birth.

Some mothers touch the baby's head or body as it emerges. The mother may glow with joy or withdraw her hand in surprise if it doesn't feel the way she expected it to.

After the birth, it may take her a few moments to realize that labor is over (or nearly so), and to shift her attention to the baby. This may take longer for some women than others.

What Does the Caregiver Do? During the crowning and birth phase, the caregiver

- Supports the mother's perineum and controls the passage of the baby's head as it crowns.
- Asks the mother to stop pushing as the head emerges. In fact, the mother should stop pushing whenever she begins to feel the burning and stretching. To do this, the mother raises her chin and blows lightly throughout the contraction. (See "Avoiding Forceful Pushing," page 109.) The uterus will still contract and give the mother an urge to push, but the mother can keep from holding her breath and straining.
- Decides if it is necessary to perform an episiotomy (see "Episiotomy," page 195).
- Holds the baby's head as it emerges and may encourage both you and the mother to touch the baby or even hold her as she comes out.
- Dries the baby and places her on the mother's abdomen where the mother can hold her, or in a heated crib nearby. A nurse or doctor checks the baby quickly and gives her an Apgar score (see page 175) when she is 1 minute old and again when she is 5 minutes old. Five signs are evaluated in order to decide if the baby needs extra immediate care, close

observation, or no extra attention at all. A total score of 7 points or above is very good. If the score is below 7, at both 1 and 5 minutes, the baby needs extra observation and care until the problems are corrected.

How Might You Feel?

- The suspense mounts as the baby's head becomes more and more visible.
- You may be barely able to contain your excitement.
- You may feel more love and awe for the mother than you ever thought possible.
- Or you may feel stunned or even queasy with so much going on at once.

How Can You Help? During the crowning and birth phase, you can help the mother in the following ways:

- Stay close by.
- If the mother is overly anxious to push the baby out and wants to push hard, give her very firm guidance to help her stop pushing so that she will not injure herself or the baby with an unduly rapid delivery.
- Help her avoid pushing by getting her to follow directions: "Raise your chin, look at me, blow . . . , blow . . . , that's the way . . . , blow . . . ," and so forth.
- Help her interpret the caregiver's directions if she is unsure about what to do.
- Remind her to look in the mirror (to see the baby's head crown and to see the baby being born) and to touch the baby's head, especially if she has said earlier that she wants to do these things. But do not be surprised or upset if she refuses. She may be unable to take in more than she is already experiencing.
- Participate in this miracle in the way that is most comfortable for you. Stay at the mother's head and focus on her if you feel squeamish about watching the baby come out. Or, take it all in by watching in the mirror or by moving so that you can watch closely. Please, though, don't get so caught up in the birth that you ignore the mother!
- Remember that although the baby's initial appearance may

be dusky (bluish) and almost lifeless, it will begin to change within seconds as the baby breathes and cries.

The Placental Stage

What Is It? The placental stage begins when the baby is born and ends after the placenta, or afterbirth, is born.

This stage is usually anticlimactic when compared with the baby's birth, and many women barely notice their few contractions and the emergence of the placenta. The two phases of the placental stage, the separation of the placenta and the expulsion of the placenta, are usually imperceptible to the mother. Medical professionals call this the *third stage* of labor.

How Long Does It Last? The placental stage is the shortest stage of labor. It usually lasts only 15 to 30 minutes.

What Does the Mother Feel? A flood of deep emotions sweeps over the mother during the placental stage. The apparent end of labor, the new baby, the rest of the job to be done—all vie for her attention.

- The mother may find the birth of the placenta interesting and fascinating, or she may devote all of her attention to the baby and you, hardly noticing when the placenta comes out.
- For a few minutes she may be unable to feel anything except relief that her ordeal is over: the pushing, the pain, the contractions have stopped.
- She may marvel at her new shape and her very soft abdomen.
- She may become preoccupied with the baby or with establishing suckling at the breast.
- She may begin to tremble all over and feel weak.

What Does the Caregiver Do? During the placental stage the caregiver

- Attends to the umbilical cord, clamping it, cutting it, or inviting you to cut it. Sometimes the caregiver withdraws some blood from the cord, to analyze for the baby's blood type or to store in a blood bank. Umbilical cord blood is a rich source of stem cells that can be used for children or adults with certain cancer or blood disorders, as an alternative to a bone marrow transplant (consult your caregiver to learn more about this procedure).

- Dries and checks the baby.
- Checks the mother's birth canal for tears.
- Attends to the placenta. When the placenta has separated from the uterine wall (the caregiver can tell by feeling the uterus and pulling gently on the cord), he or she may ask the mother to push gently to deliver the placenta.
- Carefully inspects the placenta to be sure that all of it was delivered.

How Might You Feel? At this time you will probably be engrossed with the baby and mother, and letting out your emotions—pride, joy, relief, love. You may find yourself weeping with joy and relief and showering kisses on the mother and baby.

How Can You Help? During the placental stage you can do the following:

- Cut the cord, if you want to. The symbolism of separating mother and baby appeals to some women and their partners. The cord is very firm and slippery. When you cut it, don't snip gently. It takes a decisive effort.
- Enjoy the baby and help the mother to do the same—this is your main role now. Make sure the mother is comfortable, that she can see the baby, and that she is warm enough.
- Make sure the baby stays warm. Cover her with warm blankets; don't unwrap her; keep her head covered. If a newborn is chilled, she can take a long time to regain her temperature.
- Go along if the baby has to be removed to the nursery (either because of a health problem or because it is hospital policy), unless the mother needs you to remain with her.
- Take advantage of any chance you have to hold the baby close; talk to the baby and begin getting acquainted.
- Congratulate yourselves on a job well done, and start making those phone calls, as the after-birth care (page 271) of mother and baby begins.

Normal Labor—in a Nutshell

The following table summarizes the events in normal labor and the ways you can help. You may find this table useful as a quick reference during labor.

NORMAL LABOR—IN A NUTSHELL

Stage/Phase of Labor	What Happens	How You Can Help
PRELABOR (**off-and-on or constant for hours or days**)	• The cervix softens, thins, and moves forward. • The mother has some possible or preliminary signs of labor (page 45), or both. • The mother may become anxious, discouraged, or tired if it lasts a long time.	• Encourage normal activities in the daytime, as long as they are not strenuous; rest at night. • Distracting activities are appropriate. • The mother should eat whenever she feels like it. • Time the contractions off and on. Use the "Early Labor Record" (page 54). • Be patient; do not get overexcited or preoccupied with the contractions. • The mother can use music, massage, or a shower to relax.
DILATION (FIRST) STAGE (2 to 24 hours)		
Early labor (a few hours to 20 hours)	• The cervix continues thinning, and opens to about 4 or 5 cm. • The mother has one or both positive signs of labor (page 45). Progress usually begins slowly.	• Continue as in prelabor. • Suggest a ritual of slow breathing and relaxation when the mother cannot walk or talk through contractions without pausing. • If the bag of waters breaks, take precautions (page 48); call the caregiver. • Remain with the mother, and encourage her. • Do not ask questions during contractions.

NORMAL LABOR—IN A NUTSHELL

Stage/Phase of Labor	What Happens	How You Can Help
Active labor (½ hour to 6 hours)	• The cervix dilates from about 5 to 8 cm. • Contractions become intense or painful, last 60 seconds or more, and come closer—every 4 minutes or less. • Progress speeds up. • The mother may feel trapped and discouraged; she becomes quiet, serious, and focused on her labor. • The pain of the contractions peaks by 7 or 8 cm of dilation.	• Go to the hospital, or make sure the midwife is on her way to your home. • Present the mother's Birth Plan to the nurse or midwife (page 25). • Give the mother your total, undivided attention for every contraction. • Match her quiet, serious, focused mood. • Encourage her. Point out the more rapid progress. • Use comfort measures (page 95). For backache, use cold or heat, counterpressure, positions (page 152). Use "The Take-Charge Routine" if necessary (page 134). Suggest a long bath in warm water. • If you are worried or uncertain, ask staff or caregiver for help, explanations, reassurance. • Offer a sip of liquid after each contraction. • Remind her to urinate every hour or two.
Transition phase (10 to 60 minutes)	• The cervix dilates from about 8 cm to complete (10 cm). This usually takes 5 to 20 contractions, but the presence of a cervical lip (see page 73) may prolong this phase. • The mother has long, painful contractions, with little break between. • The baby may begin descending, causing pressure in the mother's rectum and, possibly, the urge to push.	• Continue the same rituals as in the active phase. • Stay very close. • Focus on one contraction at a time. • Let the mother doze or relax between contractions. It is okay if she does not relax *during* these contractions. • Remind the mother that transition is short, that she is almost ready to begin pushing her baby out.

90

Stage/Phase of Labor	What Happens	How You Can Help
Transition phase— *continued*	• The mother becomes restless, tense, overwhelmed, irritable, despairing. She may weep, cry out, want to give up or fight contractions. She may doze during the few seconds between contractions. • The mother may tremble and vomit; her skin may hurt when rubbed.	• Use "The Take-Charge Routine" (page 134), if necessary; talk her through contractions. • A firm touch usually helps; rubbing or touching may be annoying. • Call the nurse or caregiver if the mother begins pushing. • Help her push or keep from pushing (page 104) according to the advice of the caregiver or nurse.
BIRTHING (SECOND) STAGE (15 minutes to over 3 hours)		
Resting phase (0 to 20 minutes)	• The baby's head may be in the birth canal. • The cervix is fully dilated. • The contractions may subside or seem to stop for 15 to 20 minutes. • The uterus is "catching up" with the baby. • The resting phase may not occur if the baby is very low. • The mother becomes clear-headed, optimistic, and determined. She may wonder why labor has "stopped." • The staff may want the mother to begin pushing even without contractions.	• Be patient; remind the mother of the lull of the resting phase. • If a staff member tells the mother to push without the urge, ask if she can wait for the urge to push. • Encourage the mother to relax and take advantage of the rest. • If 20 minutes pass without pushing contractions, suggest that mother change position. Try hands and knees, squatting, a supported squat, or standing (see page 112).

NORMAL LABOR—IN A NUTSHELL—*Continued*

Stage/Phase of Labor	What Happens	How You Can Help
Descent phase (10 minutes to 2½ hours)	• Strong contractions resume. • The baby moves down the birth canal. • The urge to push becomes stronger and more frequent with each contraction. • The mother cannot avoid pushing. The urge is strong and involuntary; it comes from inside. She cannot make the urge happen, although she can push without the urge. • The mother may be alarmed at feeling the baby's head in her vagina. She may "hold back" by tensing her pelvic floor. • The baby moves down during each pushing effort, and slips back between pushes.	• Remind the mother to relax her pelvic floor. Say, for example, "Open up," or "Let the baby come." • Encourage the mother to bear down and push when she feels the urge. • Suggest that the mother sit on the toilet for a few contractions if she seems to be holding back. • Hot compresses may help relax her perineum. • Reinforce her efforts. Tell her how well she is doing. • Suggest that she touch baby's head (she may or may not want to do so). • The baby's head appears wrinkled; do not be alarmed. • Help the mother change positions (see page 111) if she needs to.
Crowning and birth phase (2 to 20 minutes)	• The baby's head no longer slips back between pushes. • The birth of the head is imminent (it will emerge within a few contractions). • The mother feels an intense burning, stinging in her vagina ("the rim of fire"). She may be confused, wanting to push very hard to get the baby out right away but feeling she may split if she pushes. • The baby's head emerges, and rotates; then the shoulders and the rest of the body are born.	• Don't rush the mother; remind her to *stop pushing* and "breathe her baby out," or pant (with her chin up) to keep from pushing (page 109). • Help her tune in to the caregiver's instructions. • Help the mother hold the baby, preferably skin to skin. • Keep the baby warm; cover him with blankets.

Stage/Phase of Labor	What Happens	How You Can Help
PLACENTAL (THIRD) STAGE (5 to 30 minutes)	• The mother may be very shaky. • Her uterus cramps. • The placenta separates from wall of uterus. • The cord is clamped and cut. • The mother may hardly notice the expulsion of the placenta.	• Enjoy the baby. • Cut the cord, if you like. • Make sure the mother and baby are warm and comfortable. • Hold the baby if the mother is not ready or has pain during contractions or stitching.

NORMAL LABOR—IN A NUTSHELL

4

Comfort Measures
for Labor

*T*he pain of labor has many causes. In the first stage, pain is caused by

- Contractions of the uterus (the strongest muscle in the human body) which reach maximum intensity during this stage. (Try doing several chin-ups for a minute at a time. The muscle pain in your arms is similar to the pain of uterine contractions.)
- Stretching of the cervix as it opens. (Try sitting on the floor with your legs out straight, and bending forward as far as possible with your hands grasping your lower legs. This will give you a sense of the nature of the pain caused by the cervix stretching.)
- Stretching of pelvic ligaments, from the pressure of the baby's head within the pelvis. This causes mild to severe back pain. One-fourth to one-third of laboring women have back pain during labor.

In the second stage, pain is caused by uterine contractions, pressure in the pelvis, and also by stretching of the muscles of the pelvic floor, the vaginal canal, and the skin of the vaginal outlet.

Factors that Increase or Decrease the Pain of Labor

Labor pain can be eased or worsened by numerous physical, psychological, social, and environmental factors. A woman experiences greater pain when she feels afraid (of pain, birth, or hospitals), anxious that something is wrong, helpless, or embarrassed over her behavior or appearance. Her pain is also likely to be worse if she lacks understanding of the birth process and the reasons for the procedures and practices commonly used in the hospital. Frequent disturbances—as staff people, most of whom are strangers, come and go, ask questions, or adjust equipment—can increase pain, as can restrictions on the laboring woman's movements, sounds, or other spontaneous coping techniques. Lastly, of course, exhaustion, discouragement, hopelessness, and being left alone can add to a woman's pain.

When a laboring woman knows how to help herself and feels well cared for, her pain tends to be more manageable, and her need for pain medication is less. A woman generally experiences less pain when she understands the birth process and agrees with the use of the usual procedures; when the birth environment is comfortable, calming, and free from disturbances; when she feels respected and cared for by her support team and the staff; when she is reassured that the sensations of labor are normal; and when she is encouraged to use her self-help comfort measures.

There are many things a woman and her partner can do to reduce labor pain. Through childbirth education (classes, books, videotapes, and internet resources), they can learn about the birth process, self-help comfort measures, and choices regarding the mother's care in labor. The laboring woman can use relaxation techniques, rhythmic breathing or moaning, attention focusing, movements, and positions. The birth partner can help by never leaving the laboring woman alone; by attending to her emotional needs; by comforting her with massage, pressure, hot packs, or cold packs; by suggesting a shower or bath; and by assisting her in the use of self-help comfort measures.

This chapter will tell you more specifically what you can do to help ease the mother's pain in labor. There are numerous techniques for managing pain in labor. They do not take away *all* pain, but when combined with caring and skilled labor support, these techniques enable many women to cope successfully with their pain. Some women use these techniques in combination with pain-relieving medications; others rely totally on the techniques.

Be sure, before labor begins, that you know and respect the mother's preferences regarding her use of pain medications. Use the "Pain Medications Preference Scale," page 249, to help find out how she feels and whether your feelings are different from hers. Then you will know how to react if and when she approaches the limits of her tolerance of pain. You will either (1) ask for pain medication (see "Medications for Pain During Labor," page 225), or (2) redouble your efforts in encouraging, guiding, and helping the mother to continue handling her pain. For the latter, you will find many of the comfort measures described here to be highly effective.

The techniques described in this chapter work in any of three different ways:

- By actually eliminating or reducing factors causing the pain.
- By increasing other pleasant or neutral sensations to dampen the mother's awareness of the pain.
- By involving her in activities that focus her attention on something besides the pain.

Learn about the following techniques before labor begins so that you will be better prepared to help the mother use them. Alternating among a variety of techniques seems more helpful than doing the same thing for the entire labor. Use the information in this chapter and the lists in chapter 1 to pack a bag of comfort items to take to the hospital (or to have ready in your home) to use during labor.

The Three Rs:
Relaxation, Rhythm, and Ritual

Coping well with the pain and indeterminate length of labor involves the use of the Three Rs—relaxation, rhythm, and ritual. When a contraction begins, the woman begins her ritual, which she continues until the contraction ends. She does not use her ritual until her contractions are intense enough that she is no longer able to continue walking, talking, or doing anything through them. Rather, she pauses in her activity or stops talking during the peak of the contraction, and resumes once the peak is passed.

In early labor her ritual is usually one she has learned in advance, perhaps in childbirth class. Or a nurse or doula may teach it to her at the time. This "prescribed ritual" involves breathing slowly and rhythmically (like sighing), releasing muscle tension with each outward breath and focusing her attention in some positive way.

In active labor a woman may adopt another prescribed ritual. She may change to a light rhythmic breathing pattern, move rhythmically (sway, rock, slow-dance with her partner [page 112] or tap or stroke herself, her partner, or her pillow or another object), and focus her attention by staring into her partner's face, counting her breaths, using guided imagery, singing, moaning, or silently talking to herself. By this time in labor, however, many women stop thinking, give up the prescribed ritual, and "go on automatic." They discover their own personal, spontaneous rituals, which become very powerful aids in getting through each contraction. Once women discover these rituals, they repeat them for many contractions; then, as labor changes, they change rituals once again.

What do labor rituals have in common? They always seem to involve rhythm in some way—rocking, swaying, head movements, tapping, stroking (herself, someone else, or something); moaning, repeating a few words, or silently reciting a song, a verse, or a mantra that sticks in her mind; or visualizing a metaphor for the contraction. Sometimes the rhythm is supplied by someone or something else, in the form of murmuring, rhythmic stroking or squeezing, pouring water over her belly, or moaning or swaying with her. When a woman finds a ritual, it means she has found a way to deal with the contraction pain. If anyone disturbs her ritual, she becomes more aware of the pain, and it might take her a while to find her way back to her ritual.

Internal and External Rituals

Some women close their eyes and become very still during contractions. Their ritual is internal; it involves relaxation, rhythmic breathing, and a mental activity. Others keep their eyes open and focused, move their bodies, vocalize rhythmically, and depend on someone else to be a part of the ritual. These are external rituals, in which a woman receives help from outside herself. It is quite common for a woman to use an internal ritual early in labor and shift to an external one later, or vice versa.

How to Help with Labor Rituals

As birth partner, you can help a laboring woman develop or continue her ritual. First, observe her behavior during contractions. Is she remaining still, with relaxed muscles? Or is she moving or vocalizing? Is there rhythm in what she is doing? If she is doing any of these, she is coping well. If not, you may need to help her find or regain a ritual (see "The Take-Charge Routine," page 134). Do not interrupt her ritual during a contraction by asking a question, or telling her to try something else.

Your assistance will probably be more active when she uses an external ritual than when she uses an internal ritual. For example, with an external ritual you might

- Maintain eye-to-eye contact with her.
- Help her keep her rhythm with head or hand movements, stroke her, or talk to her in the rhythm of her breathing or moaning.
- Press firmly on her upper arms, hands, thighs, or feet to anchor her.
- Press her hips or low back (see "Counterpressure to Relieve Back Pain," page 127).
- Hold her close, walk, sway, or slow-dance with her.

If she uses an internal ritual, you might

- Remain close by, holding her hand quietly and calmly.
- Refrain from and ask others to refrain from disturbing her during contractions.

If you have prepared yourself for a very active support role, you may feel useless if the mother uses an internal ritual. You may want to do more, to have her look at you, or allow you to stroke her or talk to her. You must realize, however, that she still needs you, but for your calm, caring presence. If she is coping (relaxing during contractions and remaining still, with eyes closed), you would disturb her if you tried to get her to look at you or follow your rhythm.

However, you should continue to observe her during contractions. If she begins to wince or tense or vocalize or loses her rhythm, then you should help her regain a ritual.

Once a woman's cervix has dilated completely and she is in the second stage, she becomes more alert and focused. She is less likely to have a ritual now. The powerful contractions dictate whether, when, and how she pushes, and she approaches birth in a crescendo of emotion, excitement, and sensation. Instead of trying to help her maintain a ritual, help her maintain a good position for birth and encourage her to relax her perineum as she pushes.

The problem may be continual interruptions—a nurse or caregiver examining her, checking her pulse, taking her temperature or blood pressure, drawing blood, monitoring her, and so forth. If the mother finds interventions to be unsettling, you might say, "If we could try a few without interruption, I think she could get back on top of these contractions. Is this possible?" If the procedures cannot be postponed, you may need to play a more active "coaching" role (see "The Take-Charge Routine," page 134) until the mother can have some quiet, undisturbed time to develop her ritual.

Examples of Spontaneous Rituals

The following examples describe some spontaneous rituals developed by women and their birth partners. You can see how people add their personal touches to get the most out of the comfort measures.

One couple found themselves handling the contractions with the birth partner (her husband) scratching the mother's back during each contraction while she knelt on the floor and leaned forward onto his lap. The mother had always loved having her back scratched, and found that during contractions it really helped if he scratched it lightly, moving gradually upward from the left buttock to the left shoulder, over to the right shoulder, and down to the right buttock. Following the changes in her breathing, he timed it so that when he reached her right shoulder the contraction had peaked, and when he reached her right buttock it had ended. This back scratching was a helpful focus for the mother; she knew where she was in the contraction by where her birth partner was scratching! Later she said, "He cut my contractions in half! I knew I just had to cope until he got to my right shoulder. Then I knew I was on my way out of the contraction." Other birth partners have helped mothers know when a contraction has passed the halfway point by counting breaths (once you know about how many breaths it takes the mother to get through a contraction, you can tell her when she is "on the downside"), by calling off 10- or 15-second intervals during each contraction, or by watching the fetal monitor for signs that the contraction is fading.

In another case, the ritual involved hair brushing. The laboring woman had long, straight, silky hair, and she found that she could cope well as long as her mother brushed it rhythmically during the contractions. If her mother stopped, the woman felt more pain. It happened that her mother had often brushed the woman's hair when she was a child and teenager, and during those times they had felt very close to each other. The daughter had felt safe and content then, and these same feelings surfaced during her labor.

One woman, who was sitting up in bed with a sheet covering her legs, discovered that it really helped if her husband lightly stroked her lower leg (through the sheet) in the same rhythm as her breathing. He did this contraction after contraction. The nurse came in and did a vaginal exam to check for dilation. She removed the sheet, and, as often happens, the exam brought on a contraction. The partner, eager to help as he had been doing, began to stroke the woman's lower leg without the sheet covering it. For the woman, this was *not* her ritual. She cried out, "The sheet! The sheet!" Thus chastened, her poor partner threw the sheet over her legs and tried to get back to the old rhythm. This illustrates how important a seemingly trivial detail can be to a woman's ritual.

Another example of the importance of detail is the woman who found herself staring at a hole in her husband's tee shirt during every contraction, and repeating to herself, "Blow through the hole and you're in control. Blow through the hole and you're in control." When her husband turned away to get a drink of water during a contraction, she fell apart. She said, "You can't do that!" He thought she meant he couldn't drink water. He had no idea how important the hole in his tee shirt was!

Here is one last heartwarming ritual. A laboring woman and her partner would pace slowly between contractions, and when a contraction began they would face each other and "slow dance" (see page 112). They would sway together silently, and then resume the pacing when the contraction ended. Later, at the childbirth class reunion, he described this ritual with tears in his eyes: "I've never felt so manly in all my life. Holding her close, I could feel every contraction while she pressed against me."

The development of rituals is a truly creative aspect of labor, although it is largely unrecognized by caregivers and by childbirth educators and authors. It is not comfort measures by themselves that reduce pain; rather it is the mother's unique adaptation of these measures to suit her personality and her needs at the time.

Self-Help Comfort Measures

Relaxation

Relaxation, patterned breathing, and attention focusing have long been the cornerstones of childbirth preparation. Of these three, relaxation is the most important; it is the goal of most comfort measures. If a woman lets her body go limp during her contractions, she will feel less pain. The mother's attempt to relax, even if not completely successful, is helpful in itself because it serves as a positive focus away from her pain.

In active labor, relaxation during contractions may be harder than it was in early labor; the mother may need to keep moving. At this phase her goal should be to relax between contractions, and carry on a ritual (see page 98) during them.

During the last weeks of pregnancy, help the mother learn to recognize and release tension in all parts of her body. By practicing with her, you can learn what tone of voice, which words, and what sort of touch help her relax. Try the following:

1. While she lies still, tell the mother which parts to focus on

and relax. Start at her toes, and gradually go through her body parts to her head.

2. Help her to relax during activity—to relax parts of her body, that is, while others are tense or working. For example, you can tell her to relax her shoulders while eating, or relax her brow while watching TV. With your help she may become more aware of her tension and learn to relax those parts not needed for a particular activity.

3. If she has a "tension spot"—a part of her body where tension seems to settle whenever she is stressed—this same spot is likely to be the seat of tension during labor. Her tension spot might be in her shoulders, neck, brow, jaw, or low back. Help her identify the spot and let go of tension there when you touch it or when you say, for example, "Relax your right shoulder." If the mother has difficulty relaxing, she can learn to let a particular part of her body go limp by first tensing it (tightening the muscles as much as possible) and then relaxing it. Repeating this exercise trains the mother to recognize when her body is tense and to relax it.

4. Try "floating" an arm or leg. While the mother sits or lies comfortably, gently lift her arm, with one of your hands just above her wrist and the other beneath her elbow. Gently move her arm up and down and around in circles. Encourage her to "let go" and not help or resist your movements. Try the same thing with a leg. This exercise teaches trust as well as the difference between tension and relaxation.

Good childbirth preparation classes emphasize relaxation techniques. Audio and video tapes are also available to help people master the art of relaxation. See "Recommended Resources" for a description of tapes that I have made for pregnant women.

During labor you can help the mother to relax in the following ways:

- When she feels a contraction begin, remind her to begin her ritual immediately, releasing the tension everywhere as she breathes out.
- If she tenses in any parts of her body as the contraction intensifies, remind her with soothing words and touch to let go of the tension in those places. Don't just say, "Relax." She needs

you to be more specific than that. Instead say, "Let go right here," as you touch her hands, brow, shoulders, and so forth.

- Try "floating" a limb between contractions, if she has found this helpful.
- Use the comfort measures in this chapter and verbal reminders to help the mother relax during and between contractions. Trial and error will tell you what works best. Once you find something that works, stick with it.
- If labor becomes so intense that the mother is unable to relax *during* contractions despite your efforts, then help her relax and rest *between* contractions. Use soothing words, touch, and other comfort measures.

Hypnosis

Many laboring women can achieve a trance state during which they are able to remain relaxed, with a reduced awareness of the pain. The use of hypnosis during labor requires *proper training in advance*. The hypnotic trance can be induced by the mother herself, by a trained birth partner, or by a hypnotherapist who accompanies the mother during labor.

"Hypnobirthing" classes are popular adjuncts to conventional childbirth education. Certified hypnotherapists with special additional training work intensively with mothers and their partners, using hypnosis to reduce fear and anxiety, build confidence, and foster mastery of pain-relief techniques (see "Recommended Resources").

Attention Focusing

This technique diverts the mother's mind from her pain by having her concentrate on something else. During contractions the mother can focus her attention in one of several ways:

- She can *look* at you or at a meaningful picture or figurine, flowers, or another object. One woman hung a baby's outfit on the wall, and focused on it and the fact that she soon would fill the suit with a baby.
- She can *listen* to your voice, to music, or to another soothing sound. Many women like to hear rhythmic murmuring with each contraction.

- She can *focus* on your touch, your massage, or your caress.
- She can *concentrate* on a mental drill such as counting breaths or repeating words to herself throughout each contraction. For example, she might chant, "Ooopen . . . , ooopen . . . , ooopen . . . ," say, "I think I can . . . , I think I can . . . , I thought I could . . . , I thought I could . . . . (from *The Little Engine That Could*), or repeat, as one woman did, "Be still like the mountain and flow like the river."

Visualization

The mother can visualize something positive, pleasant, or relaxing, using her contractions, her focus, or her breathing as a cue. For example, she might visualize her exhalations or your soothing touch or massage as drawing her tension and pain away. She might visualize each contraction in various ways: as a wave, with herself floating over the crest; or as a mountain, which she climbs up and down as the contractions come and go. She might use the onset of the contraction as a cue to imagine herself soaring like a seagull above the waves of contractions below. Several women from my childbirth classes have told me that during labor they visualized the opening of the cervix of my knitted argyle uterus, which I have used to demonstrate contractions and dilation during classes. Some visualizations are planned; others emerge spontaneously in labor. They are usually very creative and personally helpful.

Rhythmic Breathing and Moaning Patterns

Breathing patterns, along with relaxation, have represented the mainstay of childbirth preparation since its inception. Although some childbirth educators have abandoned patterned breathing because it keeps the mother from behaving spontaneously during labor, I think it has tremendous value because it offers the following unique pain-relieving capabilities:

- Patterned breathing helps the mother relax, especially when she has learned to release tension each time she breathes out.
- Patterned breathing, with its steady rhythm, is calming, especially when labor is in turmoil.

- Patterned breathing may give the mother a sense of well-being, letting her know she has some measure of control over her own behavior, even though her uterus, with its involuntary and all-encompassing contractions, is completely outside her conscious control.
- When institutional policies or the woman's own condition does not permit a wide range of behavior, patterned breathing is always available as an effective comfort measure. For example, the mother may not be able to use some of the other comfort measures, such as baths or showers and movement, because (1) she cannot get out of bed, (2) an electronic fetal monitor or intravenous line is in the way, or (3) she has received medications that make using these comfort measures impossible. (See "When the Mother Must Labor in Bed," page 158, for specific suggestions for such circumstances.)

The mother should learn and practice the various breathing patterns before labor so that she will be able to use them most effectively and with the least effort during labor—when she will really need them.

Breathing Patterns for Labor. There are two basic breathing patterns for the dilation (first) stage: slow breathing and light breathing. I suggest that you and the mother learn each of these, adapt their speed and rhythm so you feel comfortable with them, and then use them as you like during labor. The mother's preferences and the nature of the contractions should guide the two of you in deciding how and when to use the patterns.

Because slow breathing is easiest and most relaxing, I usually suggest beginning with it as part of the mother's ritual for active labor (distracting activities should help her cope with early labor). She starts when the contractions reach a level of intensity at which she cannot continue walking, or talking, or whatever she is doing, right through the contraction—in other words, when she has to pause until the contraction eases. From this point on she should continue with slow breathing for as long as she can relax well with it, perhaps moaning or sighing audibly with each outward breath.

Slow Breathing. Slow breathing is very relaxing and calming. The key is that the mother breathe easily and not work too hard to keep it slow: "Easy in, easy out." If she is working too hard, her breathing will sound tense and strained. This is how to use slow breathing during labor:

1. When the contraction begins, the mother focuses her attention, as described on page 104.
2. She takes a big, relaxing sigh, releasing tension throughout her body as she breathes out.
3. She breathes slowly in through her nose and—preferably, though not absolutely necessarily—out through her mouth, in long breaths, with each outward breath sounding like a sigh. The rate is somewhere between 5 and 12 breaths a minute.
4. With each outward breath she relaxes, releasing tension from one part of her body.
5. As the contraction ends, her last breath is the "goodbye" breath. It is one less contraction that she must get through.

The mother should use slow breathing for as long as it continues to help her relax. Some women use only slow breathing throughout labor; others use it until the cervix opens to 6 to 8 centimeters; still others, with very intense, close contractions, may get relief by switching to light breathing even earlier. If the mother switches to light breathing early in labor, she might be able to return to slow breathing after a while. Suggest this, because slow breathing is restful and light breathing may be tiring.

Light Breathing. The light breathing pattern takes some practice to learn, just as it takes time to learn to breathe rhythmically while swimming the crawl stroke. And, just as rhythmic breathing when swimming enables one to swim better, the light breathing pattern enables the mother to better manage pain. This is how to use light breathing during labor:

1. When the contraction begins, the mother focuses her attention.
2. She begins breathing in short, light breaths through her mouth, with a silent in-breath and an audible out-breath, at a rate of 30 to 60 breaths per minute.

3. She continues at this rate until the contraction begins to subside. Then she slows down her breathing rate, if she wishes, or continues at the same rate until the contraction is over.

4. When the contraction ends, she rests or resumes whatever she was doing before it started.

Please encourage the mother to practice this pattern enough to master it. It doesn't take more than a few practice sessions. At first light breathing is uncomfortable (it may cause dry mouth, lightheadedness, or a feeling that she can't get enough air), but by adapting it and working with it, she can learn to remain relaxed and comfortable while doing it. Light breathing may become her best friend in labor (besides you).

Practice this pattern until the mother is able to do the peak rate of 30 to 60 breaths per minute for a full 1½ to 2 minutes without stopping or feeling lightheaded (from hyperventilating). If she feels lightheaded, have her slow her pace slightly or breathe more shallowly. The lightheadedness is harmless, although it is annoying and uncomfortable; it will not occur once she masters the technique. See that the mother relaxes all over, especially in the shoulders and trunk, as she practices this pattern. If she is tense, she is more likely to hyperventilate. Remind her to relax. Pace the mother by breathing with her or by using your hand to "conduct" her breathing. Keep your hand and wrist relaxed and floppy while conducting. Your own relaxation is contagious and will help her relax.

The mother should feel free to adapt these breathing patterns during labor in whatever way makes her comfortable. She may want to combine slow and light breathing; for example, she might begin and end the contraction with slow breathing and use light breathing over the peak.

Or she may like the pant-pant-blow pattern, as follows:

1. Through her mouth, she takes three or four short, light, panting breaths in and out, followed by a *long*, slow, relaxing breath out. She emphasizes each out-breath, making it audible, or even moaning through it. In-breaths are silent.

2. She repeats this short-short-short-short-long ("pant-pant-blow") pattern until the end of the contraction, when she relaxes until the next one.

Do remember, however, that breathing patterns are beneficial only if the mother can use them easily—without thinking much about them, without discomfort, and without tensing. These patterns should be relaxing; they become good attention-focusing aids in themselves once the mother has practiced them.

Breathing Patterns for Pushing (Bearing-Down Techniques). There are three techniques for handling the urge to push: One is used to *avoid forceful pushing* (or bearing down) when this would be nonproductive or harmful. The others are used during the birthing stage, when the mother *should* be pushing; they are *spontaneous bearing down, self-directed pushing*, and *directed pushing*.

Avoiding Forceful Pushing. There are two occasions during labor when the mother might feel like pushing (holding her breath and straining) but should not do so:

- During transition she may have a strong urge to push while there is still a firm lip, or rim, of cervix remaining. Forceful pushing might cause swelling of the cervix from the increased pressure of the baby against it, thus slowing the progress of labor. Until the lip has disappeared, the mother should push only enough to satisfy her urge. This "grunt pushing" helps to keep her from straining too hard. (See "Transition," page 73.)
- During the birthing stage, as the baby's head crowns and emerges, pushing hard might cause too rapid stretching and injury to the mother's vagina, or too rapid a delivery. To help the mother avoid too rapid stretching, have her avoid holding her breath, by breathing in and out and out constantly or by raising her chin and blowing or panting lightly whenever she feels the urge to push.

Blowing or panting through the urge to push is easier said than done, because the urge can be very strong. Grunt-pushing may be easier for the mother. You might talk her through each contraction, helping her to keep breathing or do grunt-pushes.

Don't expect too much from these techniques; they do not take away or diminish the mother's urge to push. All they do is help her keep from adding to the pushing that her body is already doing.

Spontaneous Bearing Down. Once the mother feels like pushing and her cervix is fully dilated or nearly so, her caregiver will give the go-ahead. Then the mother should push spontaneously. Spontaneous bearing down works like this:

1. The contraction begins. The mother focuses her attention as described on page 104.
2. She uses whichever breathing pattern (slow or light) seems best, until her urge to push is so strong that she cannot resist bearing down.
3. The urge to push comes in waves or surges—three to six in each contraction. These surges of the uterus sweep the mother along into an involuntary bearing-down effort (holding her breath or grunting, moaning, or straining) that lasts 5 to 7 seconds.
4. The surge subsides, and she breathes lightly again until the next surge. She continues in this manner until the contraction is over.
5. The contraction ends, and she rests until the next one.

Self-Directed Pushing. This is reserved for those times when the mother is holding her breath and bearing down, but her bearing down is ineffective. Her eyes may be clenched shut and she may be arching her back, tipping her chin up (sometimes referred to as "diffuse pushing"). If she is making progress while pushing this way, do not worry. But if the baby is not coming down, try this:

1. Between contractions, tell her to keep her eyes open during the next contraction.
2. If she opens her eyes for a few seconds, then shuts them again, keep reminding her to open them.
3. Ask her to look down toward where the baby will be coming out. This will keep her focused on the direction toward which she will be pushing. Or, it may help if she looks straight at her caregiver or nurse, who stands at the foot of the bed and encourages her. You might hold a mirror where she can see it (but do not do so if there is no sign of progress!). Do not be surprised if she does not want to look. This should be her choice.
4. She should bear down spontaneously, incorporating these changes.

5. Any change of position—it hardly matters which position she uses—may help her focus better and push more effectively.

6. If these measures do not succeed, try "Directed Pushing."

Directed Pushing. Until 1980 or so, directed pushing was the only bearing-down technique used in virtually every hospital and by virtually all caregivers. Today it is used under the following circumstances:

- When the mother has epidural anesthesia and cannot fully feel the urge to push, and so cannot use the spontaneous bearing-down pattern.
- When the baby's descent is too slow with spontaneous bearing down and the caregiver is considering assisting the delivery with instruments—forceps or vacuum extractor (see pages 197 to 200).
- When directed pushing remains the routine in the institution. Ask the mother's caregiver in advance whether the staff advocates spontaneous bearing down or directed pushing.

The directed-pushing technique works like this:

1. The contraction begins. The mother focuses.

2. She breathes in and out twice; she takes a third breath in and holds it. She holds her breath and strains (pushes) for a count to 10, then releases her breath. She takes several quick breaths in and out, and repeats the breath holding and straining. She continues in this way until the contraction subsides.

3. The contraction ends. She rests until the next one.

Movement and Position Changes

When the mother is free to move and change positions, she is more comfortable, and her labor may even speed up. Encourage her to try a change in position or movement if she is restless, discouraged, or in a lot of pain, or if labor has slowed down. A change every half-hour or so may make a positive difference under these circumstances. She can try standing, walking, sitting, semireclining, squatting, kneeling, lying on her side, getting on her hands and knees, or leaning on you, the wall, a birth

Position	Unique Contributions
Standing	• Takes advantage of gravity during and between contractions. • Makes contractions shorter and more productive • Helps position the fetus to enter the pelvis • May speed labor if the woman has been lying down • May increase the urge to push in the second stage
Walking*	Same as standing, plus: • Causes changes in the pelvic joints that encourage rotation and descent
Standing and leaning forward on the partner, the bed, or a birth ball*	Same as standing, plus: • Relieves backache • Makes it easy for the partner to give a back rub • May be more restful than standing upright • Can be used with an electronic fetal monitor (the mother must stand by the bed)
Slow dancing: The mother embraces her partner around the neck, and rests her head on the partner's chest or shoulder. The partner's arms are around the mother's trunk, with fingers interlocked at her low back. She drops her arms, and rests against her partner. They sway to the music, breathing in the same rhythm.*	Same as standing, plus: • Causes changes in the pelvic joints that encourage rotation and descent • Being embraced by a loved one increases the mother's sense of well-being • Rhythm and music add comfort • Pressure from the partner's hands relieves back pain
The lunge: The mother places one foot on the seat of a chair beside her, with her raised knee and foot turned out. Bending her raised knee and hip, she "lunges" sideways repeatedly during a contraction (in the direction of the fetal occiput, if she knows it, or in the direction that is more comfortable), holding the stretch for 5 seconds at a time. She should feel the stretch in her inner thighs. Secure the chair, and help her balance.*	• Widens the side of the pelvis toward which she lunges • Encourages the rotation of a baby in occiput posterior (OP) position • Can also be done in a kneeling position

* These positions are particularly helpful for back labor.

Position	Unique Contributions
Sitting upright**	• Gives the mother a rest between contractions • Uses gravity to help the baby descend • Can be used with an electronic fetal monitor
Sitting on a toilet or commode**	Same as sitting upright, plus: • May help relax the perineum for effective bearing down
Semisitting**	Same as sitting upright, plus: • Makes a vaginal exam possible • Easy position to get into on a bed or delivery table
Sitting and rocking in a chair	Same as sitting upright, plus: • May speed labor
Sitting, leaning forward with support*	Same as sitting upright, plus: • Relieves backache • Makes it easy for the partner to give a back rub
Hands-and-knees position*	• Helps relieve backache • Assists the rotation of a baby in OP position • Allows for pelvic rocking and other body movements • Makes a vaginal exam possible • Takes pressure off hemorrhoids
Kneeling, leaning forward on a chair seat, the raised head of the bed, or a birth ball*	Same as hands and knees, plus: • Puts less strain on wrists and hands
Open knee-chest position: The mother gets on hands and knees, then lowers her chest so her buttocks are higher than her chest. Be sure her knees are apart and back far enough to raise her buttocks. Let her lean against you, or hold her by the shoulders to help her maintain the position.*	• Uses gravity to promote movement of the baby's head (or buttocks) out of the pelvis, and reduces pressure on the cervix, which may be desirable if the cord is prolapsed, the cervix is swollen, or the baby is in OP position • Spending 30 to 45 minutes in this position is sometimes recommended in early labor when a baby is in OP position and contractions are frequent, very painful, and accompanied by back pain and no progress in dilation

* These positions are particularly helpful for back labor.
** These positions are useful during the birthing stage.

POSITIONS AND MOVEMENTS FOR LABOR AND BIRTH

Position	Unique Contributions
Sidelying	• Gives the mother some rest • Makes interventions easy to perform • Helps lower elevated blood pressure • Safer than standing or the hands-and-knees position if pain medications are used • May promote the progress of labor when alternated with walking • Can slow a very rapid second stage • Takes pressure off hemorrhoids • Allows relaxation between pushing efforts
Squatting**	• May relieve backache • Uses gravity to help the baby descend • May aid the baby's rotation • Widens the pelvic outlet • Provides the mechanical advantage of the upper trunk pressing on the uterus • May help bring on the urge to push • Requires less bearing-down effort • Allows freedom to shift weight for comfort
Lap squatting: Sit on an armless straight chair. The mother sits on your lap facing you, straddling your thighs. Embrace each other. When a contraction begins, spread your thighs, allowing her buttocks to sag between. After the contraction, bring your legs together so the mother is sitting on them.**	Same as squatting, plus: • Avoids the strain on the mother's knees and ankles • Allows for more support with less effort for an exhausted mother • Enhances feelings of well-being, as the mother is held close by a loved one
Supported squat: Hold the mother under the arms as she leans with her back against you during contractions, and bear all her weight. Between contractions, she stands.**	• Lengthens the mother's trunk, allowing more room for the baby to maneuver into position • Enhances pelvic joint mobility, allowing the baby to push the pelvic bones as needed to descend • Uses gravity to help the baby descend

** These positions are useful during the birthing stage.

POSITIONS AND MOVEMENTS FOR LABOR AND BIRTH

114

Position	Unique Contributions
Dangle: Sit on a high bed or counter, with your feet supported on chairs or footrests and your thighs spread. Standing, the mother backs between your legs and places her flexed arms over your thighs. Grip her chest with your thighs. During contractions she lowers herself, allowing you to support her full weight. Between contractions she stands.**	Same as supported squat, plus: • Puts much less strain on the partner

** This position is useful during the birthing stage.

ball, the bed, or the nightstand (see the illustrations on page 116). Don't insist that she change position, however, especially when she has a good ritual and is making good progress.

Some women use a series of positions with each contraction—for example, sitting or walking between contractions, then standing up and leaning on the birth partner during contractions. (See "Backache During Labor," page 150, for further discussion of the use of positions during the dilation stage.)

During the birthing stage, too, the mother may use several different positions, especially if this stage takes more than an hour. Just before the actual birth of the baby, the caregiver may ask the mother to assume a position that he or she prefers (such as semisitting). See pages 112 to 115 for a list of useful positions and the possible benefits of each.

Comfort Aids and Devices

Baths and Showers (Hydrotherapy)

One of the safest and most effective forms of pain relief in labor is immersion in deep water or a warm shower. Hydrotherapy has been used for relaxation, healing, and pain relief for centuries, and today is widely used in physical therapy, sports medicine, and other health disciplines. It has been used in child-

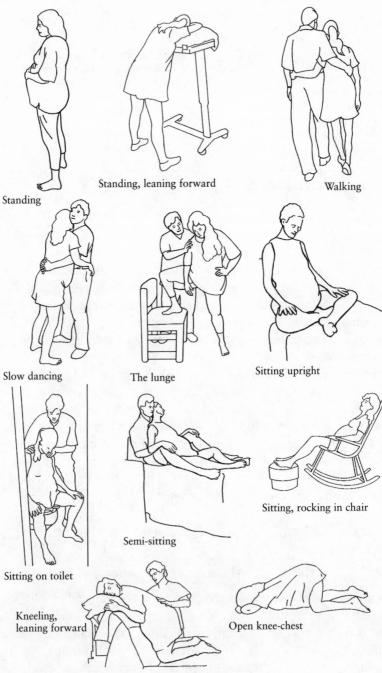

Standing

Standing, leaning forward

Walking

Slow dancing

The lunge

Sitting upright

Sitting on toilet

Semi-sitting

Sitting, rocking in chair

Kneeling, leaning forward

Open knee-chest

Positions and movements for labor and birth.

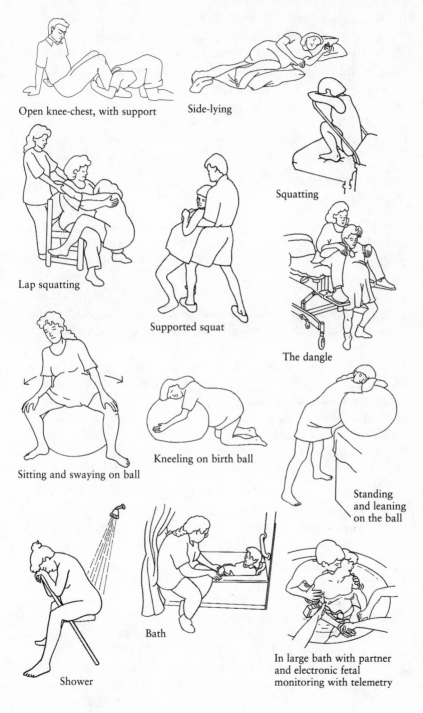

Open knee-chest, with support

Side-lying

Squatting

Lap squatting

Supported squat

The dangle

Sitting and swaying on ball

Kneeling on birth ball

Standing and leaning on the ball

Shower

Bath

In large bath with partner and electronic fetal monitoring with telemetry birth, however, only since the 1980s. Showers are available in most hospitals, and bathtubs (some large enough for the woman to move around in or to share with her partner!) have been installed in most modern hospitals. Some hospitals have tubs on wheels that can be moved from one birthing room to another. Lightweight tubs can be rented and set up temporarily in one's home for a home birth, or possibly even in a hospital, if the staff is willing and arrangements have been made in advance (see "Recommended Resources").

Most women who use water in labor use it for pain relief. Soaking in a tub or lingering in the shower is soothing and relaxing. Numerous studies have shown that hydrotherapy, when used correctly during labor, is safe, reduces pain, and frequently speeds labor. We sometimes call the bath "the midwife's epidural." Unlike with a true epidural, the mother is able to move about normally. She also remains clearheaded. Some women give birth in water. Unfortunately, this practice is restricted almost completely to out-of-hospital settings in North America, although it is supported in many European hospitals.

How Does a Bath Reduce Pain and Speed Labor? Michel Odent, M.D., has tirelessly studied the physiology of immersion in water. I summarize his explanation here, along with his recommendations for the safest and most effective use of water in labor.

When a person sits in a deep warm bath, a series of physiological changes begins immediately. These changes alter hormone production and fluid distribution throughout the body.

The laboring woman's body responds quickly to immersion:

- The warmth and buoyancy of the water bring about immediate relaxation and relief of pain. This lowers the production of stress hormones (such as adrenalin), which are known to work against oxytocin and to slow contractions.
- The body's own oxytocin (which has very different effects than the chemical form used to induce labor) is secreted by the pituitary gland in larger quantities.
- Labor progresses faster with the increase in oxytocin, without an increase in pain.
- The oxytocin causes feelings of calm and well-being (an effect that does not occur with intravenous oxytocin).

- The weight of the water (hydrostatic pressure) against the woman's tissues presses fluid from her arms, legs, and skin into her circulation, which markedly increases her blood volume, especially in her chest and heart.
- The increased fluid volume speeds kidney action, often causing an urgent need to urinate.

Long immersion in water is not beneficial. A secondary effect of the increased blood volume in the chest begins slowly, and takes a couple of hours to become obvious. The heart produces atrial natriuretic factor (ANF), which plays an important role in maintaining fluid balance. One effect of ANF is to slowly suppress the production of oxytocin. For this reason, labor tends to slow if the woman does not get out of the water after one to two hours. In fact, many women sense the change and get out of the bath on their own volition. It is wise to ask the mother to get out after about 1½ hours if she does not think to do so herself.

Although a bath frequently speeds labor for an hour or two, the effect is unlikely to continue for longer than that. Pain relief from immersion does not last for hours, either, unless the pain relief is a side effect of a slow labor.

When Should a Woman Get into the Bath? Because the beneficial effects are short-term, timing of the bath is important. If she gets in too early and stays for a long time, she will get no benefit. She should try to wait until her cervix has dilated 5 centimeters or more. Then she is likely to experience immediate and profound pain relief, along with more progress in dilation. Before this point she can take a shower, which will not cause the release of ANF.

One situation in which an earlier bath may help is when a woman is having a very long, uncomfortable prelabor or early labor. If she has missed a night's sleep with contractions, and is tired and discouraged, then she might try a long bath to stop the contractions and give her some rest.

What Water Temperature Is Best? The water temperature should be very close to body temperature, around 98.6 degrees Fahrenheit or 37 degrees Celsius. If the water is too warm, the mother's temperature will go up, the baby may develop a fever in the uterus, and the baby's heart rate might speed up too much for safety. This is very important, because a fever in the baby, even when it is not caused by infection, is serious. The baby in the uterus has no way to cool himself down. Furthermore, the mother may lose her energy if she is in too hot a tub for too long.

Is a Bath Safe if the Membranes Have Ruptured? The numerous reports in the medical literature indicate that a bath does not increase the risk of infection if a woman has ruptured membranes.

Can the Staff Monitor the Baby While the Mother Is in the Water? Yes. Waterproof hand-held monitors are available. Most midwives who attend water births outside of hospitals have these. Some hospitals also have them. If yours does not, a portable telemetry monitoring unit can be used. Someone holds the radio device out of the water, and the regular sensing device can be covered with plastic and worn in the water by the woman. If her caregiver has doubts, he or she should check with the hospital's engineering department. An engineer can confirm the safety of immersing the sensing devices.

What about Modesty? If the mother does not want to be naked, she can wear a sports bra in the water, and shorts until the birth becomes imminent. Or she can use a towel to cover exposed parts of her body. It is unlikely that she will be able to cover up completely all the time, unless she is in a conventional-size bathtub, in which a towel will probably be adequate.

What if the Baby Is Born in the Water? This is always possible; a rapid labor is not always easy to control. If the hospital has a strong policy against birth in the water, then the woman will need to be watched closely and removed in time. If the baby is born in the water, he should be immediately brought to the surface and held with his head completely out of the water. His head should be dried. Mother and baby should get out of the water before the expulsion of the placenta, because the placenta causes quite a mess if expelled in the water.

Water births happen every day, and are considered a worthy option in hospitals in the United Kingdom. There, over four thousand water births in a 25-month period were closely studied. The outcomes were excellent, and comparable to outcomes of nonwater births in which the mothers had been judged to be at very low risk of complications.

The Birth Ball

Large inflated balls made of tough vinyl are widely used in physical therapy for balance problems, back ailments, building strength and flexibility, and aiding relaxation. In childbirth, we use such a ball as a comfort device in the following ways:

- The mother sits on it and sways during contractions. This helps relax her trunk and pelvic floor. (See the illustrations on page 116.)
- The mother kneels on the floor (with padding under her knees) or bed and leans forward with her head, shoulders, arms, and upper chest resting on the ball. This provides the same benefits as the hands-and-knees position (for example, relief of back pain, rotation of an OP baby [see page 44], and possible improvement of a baby's heart rate) but is more restful. The mother can also sway effortlessly.
- The mother stands next to a birthing bed, which may be raised or lowered to a comfortable height. The ball is placed on the bed, and she rests her head and upper body on it, swaying rhythmically and effortlessly side to side during contractions. This gives many of the same advantages of kneeling over the ball, and also uses gravity to help the baby descend.
- Lastly, after the baby is born, the birth ball is a great help at home. A crying or fussy baby can almost always be quickly soothed and calmed if you or the mother sits on the ball with the baby against your shoulder. Then you bounce, gently or vigorously—whatever works. This is a wonderful way to create a soothing up-and-down motion for the baby without wearing yourself out! Of course, babies should not be bounced if their fussiness is due to hunger; they should be fed.

Birth balls come in a variety of sizes and shapes. The woman of average height (5 feet 3 inches to 5 feet 10 inches) seems to benefit most from a ball with a diameter of 65 or 75 centimeters when inflated. Shorter women do well with the 55- or 65-centimeter balls, and taller women do well with the 75- or even 85-centimeter balls. The thickness and elasticity of the vinyl vary from one brand to another, and may affect whether a particular ball will actually inflate to its stated diameter. The degree of inflation can be varied to adjust the size and firmness of the ball.

Similar inflated devices come in the shapes of huge eggs and peanuts. Such shapes make swaying more difficult, although they allow some movement. Some midwives and doulas favor them because they believe a woman is less likely to fall off one of these than a round ball.

Precautions with a Birth Ball

- If the ball is to be used on the floor, place a clean blanket or sheet on the floor beneath to keep the ball clean.
- Place a sheet, towel, or waterproof pad over the ball before the mother uses it in labor.
- Always have the mother hold onto something or someone stable as she gets situated on the ball. If she is leaning on it, hold it still.
- When she sits, remind her that her feet should remain planted on the floor, in front of the ball and about 2 feet apart. She should not straddle the ball.
- Stand close by, holding her hand, until it is clear that she is completely safe and comfortable on the ball. This takes about 1 or 2 minutes with some women, longer with others.
- When she wants to get off the ball, assist her.
- The ball should be cleaned between uses by different people. (Hospitals use the same cleaning compound that is used to clean a hospital bed.)
- Keep the ball away from sharp objects or heat sources.

Even if your hospital has birth balls, you may want to buy your own to use to soothe your baby in the months after birth. The balls costs between $25 and $50, and are available from many toy stores, department stores, and hospital physical therapy departments. Be sure that any ball you buy is intended to hold up to 300 pounds. Less expensive balls may not be sturdy enough to hold an adult.

Heat and Cold

Heat and cold can be used at any time during labor and afterwards to relieve a number of discomforts. For example

- Place a hot water bottle, a hot damp towel, or an electric heating pad on the mother's low abdomen, back, or groin to ease pain during the dilation (first) stage. (Check with the hospital before using an electric heating pad; some hospitals do not allow this.)
- Use a warm blanket to relieve trembling during the transition phase.
- Use warm compresses on the perineum (the area between her vagina and anus) during the birthing stage to relieve pain and to help her relax her birth canal.
- Use a cool damp washcloth to wipe the mother's neck, brow, and face between contractions.
- Use an ice wrap, an ice bag, a rubber glove filled with crushed ice, frozen wet washcloths, or a bag of frozen peas to relieve low back pain. Or roll an ice-filled, hollow plastic rolling pin (made by Tupperware); a can of frozen juice; or a frozen, rounded plastic bottle of water over her back.
- Use cold packs to relieve pain from hemorrhoids or stitches after the birth.

Caution: Be careful not to make the packs so hot or so cold that you cause burns or frost damage to the mother's skin. The rule is this: If you can't hold it in your hands, don't put it on her. Let the hot pack cool, or put layers of towels between her skin and the hot or cold pack to protect her, if necessary.

Transcutaneous Electrical Nerve Stimulation (TENS)

TENS has been used successfully for years to treat postoperative and chronic pain. It is now also used for childbirth and postcesarean pain. Because TENS is still unknown to many obstetric caregivers, you may have to suggest it yourself if you are interested. The mother's caregiver can obtain more information about TENS from a physical therapist.

A TENS unit is available for rent from the hospital physical therapy department or from medical-supply rental companies.

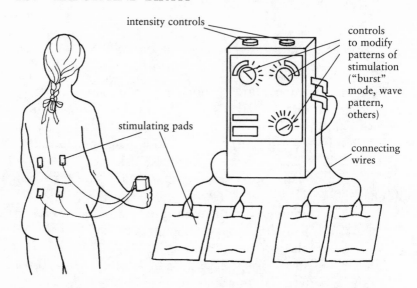

intensity controls

controls
to modify
patterns of
stimulation
("burst"
mode, wave
pattern,
others)

stimulating pads

connecting
wires

A transcutaneous electrical nerve stimulation (TENS) unit in use (left) *and a detailed look at the device* (right).

The unit consists of four flexible, Band-Aid-sized pads connected by wires to a small (cassette tape–sized) battery-operated generator of electric impulses. The pads adhere to the mother's skin alongside her low spine. You or she can regulate the impulses. During a contraction you turn on the current by turning up two dials until she feels a vibration, tingling, or prickling—just enough to diminish her awareness of the pain. When the contraction ends, you turn down the current so that she feels nothing.

Consult her caregiver if the mother wants to try TENS or to learn more about it. A physical therapist can show both of you how to use the TENS unit.

Many women who have used TENS during labor swear it enabled them to avoid using pain-relieving medication; others report TENS was helpful in diminishing their pain, especially back pain; still others say it did little good. As for safety, no adverse effects have been reported, except that TENS sometimes interferes with output from the electronic fetal monitor.

The pads should be removed if the mother wants to get into a shower or bath.

Comforting Techniques for You to Try

Touch and Massage

Touch conveys a kind, caring, and comforting message to the laboring mother. Find out what kind of touch the mother finds soothing and try it during labor. She will appreciate a gentle, comforting gesture—rubbing a painful spot, patting her reassuringly, embracing her tightly, stroking her hair or cheek. Or, she may prefer a more formal massage—a rhythmic rubbing or kneading of her back, legs, buttocks, shoulders, and so forth. Use oil or cornstarch on your hands so they won't stick to and irritate the mother's skin.

Try a very light massage (with the fingertips only—this is sometimes called *effleurage*) on the mother's abdomen during contractions. You can also use this light massage on her thighs or elsewhere if she finds it more relaxing than a firm massage. The mother may find rubbing and stroking wonderful during early labor but intolerable during transition. If so, try holding her head or shoulders, hand, foot, or thigh firmly—without rubbing.

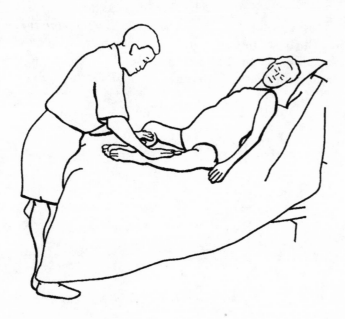

During or between contractions, try firmly squeezing and rubbing her hands and feet.

Try other ways of holding, touching, and massaging the mother, so that she can help you learn how she likes to be touched.

Acupressure. *Shiatsu*, or acupressure, has been practiced in Asia for many centuries. This healing art is derived from the ancient Chinese understanding of the principles of *yin* and *yang*. The body is made up of twelve meridians, along which vital forces flow; acupressure corrects imbalances in the flow of these vital forces. Acupressure uses the same points for stimulation as does acupuncture, but involves finger pressure instead of needles. Although these ideas are outside of Western scientific thought, the use of acupressure has gained interest in the West. Many people successfully combine acupressure with other methods to provide comfort and promote progress in labor.

By pressing with your finger or thumb at certain acupressure points, you may be able to relieve the mother's pain and speed up her labor. The two most popular points for labor are the Ho-ku point and Spleen 6. Both are sensitive spots that may hurt a bit when you press them. Your goal, however, is not to cause pain, so do not press hard enough to hurt her.

The Ho-ku point is on the back of the hand, where the bones forming the bases of the thumb and index finger come together. Press steadily into the bone at the base of the index finger with your thumb for 10 to 60 seconds, three to six times, with a rest

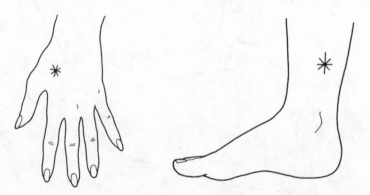

The Ho-ku point (left) and Spleen 6, four of her finger-breadths above her inner ankle bone (right).

of equal length in between. You can repeat this as often as you and the mother want.

Spleen 6 is on the inner side of the lower leg about four finger breadths above the ankle. Press your thumb into the bone from slightly behind it for 10 to 60 seconds at a time, three to six times, with a rest of equal length in between. You can repeat this whenever you and the mother want.

Caution: Experts advise against pressing these points on a pregnant woman before her due date, as they can cause contractions and increase the risk of premature labor. Find the points on yourself, but don't use them on the mother until the need arises.

Counterpressure. This is very helpful in coping with back pain. Holding the front of the mother's hip with one hand (to help her maintain balance), press steadily and firmly (with your fist or the heel of your hand) in one spot in the lower back or buttocks area. She will help you find out what spot to press—it varies from woman to woman and within the same labor. Try pressing in several places, and she will tell you when you have found the spot. You will probably have to press very hard during every contraction. Between contractions, you might massage the area or use cold or hot compresses (see page 123).

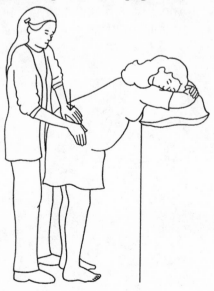

The Double Hip Squeeze. This is also helpful for back pain. The mother stands or kneels and leans forward onto a bed, birth ball, or chair seat, or gets on her hands and knees. From behind, press on both sides of her buttocks with the palms of your hands. Push toward the center, pressing her hips together. Experiment to find the right places to press. When you have found the right places, press them steadily throughout each contraction. Apply as much pressure as she needs.

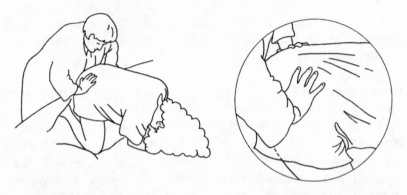

The Knee Press. This releases tension and discomfort in the low back. The mother sits upright in a chair that will not slide. You kneel on the floor in front of her, cup one hand over each of her knees, and lean toward her so that you are pressing straight back toward her hip points during each contraction.

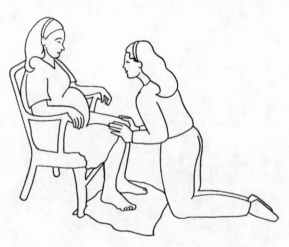

Rolling Pressure Over the Low Back. Use a rolling pin (preferably a hollow one filled with ice) or a can of frozen juice or cold soda pop (keep a six-pack in a bowl of ice, so you'll always have a cold can). Roll the pin or can over the mother's low back to soothe her during or between contractions. Since such tools are rarely available in hospitals, you might bring them in, especially if she has back labor before you leave home.

Music and Sound

Many women can relax and focus better if their favorite music or environmental sounds are played during labor. In fact, familiar and well-loved music has been found to raise levels of endorphins (the body's own pain-relieving substances). Music and environmental sounds (such as ocean waves, a babbling brook, a rain shower) create a pleasing soundscape and may overshadow some of the beeps, pages, and other sounds that are part of any modern birthing room.

You might suggest that the mother select some of her favorite recordings of music or other sounds to play during labor. Check on the availability of audio equipment in the hospital and, if necessary, bring your own.

Aromatherapy, or Pleasant Scents

Pleasant aromas create feelings of well-being and relaxation, and they cover up hospital smells. Scents such as lavender, sandalwood, lemon, and mint may appeal to the mother. You can purchase scented massage oil, bath beads, liquid soap, or cologne, or you can simply cut a lemon in half for her to sniff.

Because preferences for scents are very personal, ask the mother if she would like to have them available and, if so, which ones she would like. She may want none at all, or she may pick one or two favorites to have available during labor.

Unless a trained aromatherapist prepares special mixes for her from essential oils, stick with commercially prepared lotions and oil mixes. Essential oils are very strong, and if they are too concentrated or used incorrectly, they can cause burns, allergic reactions, and other side effects.

Taking Care of Yourself

We sometimes forget that labor can be long and tiring, stressful, and demanding for the birth partner, just as it is for the mother. Losing a night's sleep is never easy. Standing for long periods, skipping meals, and offering the mother constant optimism and encouragement are tiring, especially if you are worried or overextended. To be an effective birth partner you will need to pace yourself, draw on the experience and wisdom of others, and look after your own basic needs. This cannot mean taking long breaks for naps or meals, because the mother may need you and want you to stay. She will probably depend heavily on you to help her through every contraction. There are ways you can take care of her and of yourself at the same time. Here are some suggestions to help you conserve energy and get appropriate help from others:

- Be sure to have your supplies handy. See the list of suggested items for the birth partner's use during labor (page 15).
- Eat and drink tasty, nourishing food and beverages regularly during labor. Choose foods without strong odors, and keep them with you so you do not have to leave the room to get them.
- Wear comfortable clothes, and have a sweater and slippers available.
- Rest, by making yourself comfortable near the mother. Don't stand when you can sit. If the mother is lying down and you also need some rest, you can lie down next to her, or sit and rest your head on the bed beside her. If there is enough time between contractions, doze. You will not have trouble waking up to help her if you keep a hand on her arm or belly.
- Ask for reassurance. If you are worried about the length of labor or about the mother's pain or discouragement or fatigue, ask the caregiver or nurse if everything is all right; express your concerns. It is best, however, to do this outside the mother's hearing.
- Ask the nurse or caregiver for ideas for comfort measures. If you are uncertain whether you are helping the mother enough, ask for suggestions.

- Seek help from another support person or a doula. Many women have more than one helper; for example, a relative or friend might be present, along with the husband or lover. The two helpers can spell each other at times and work together at other times. Increasingly, women or couples request the services of a doula, who has a broader perspective on childbirth and more experience with it. A doula can raise your morale and the mother's, make concrete suggestions for comfort measures, help you remember some of the things you learned in childbirth class, and remind you and the mother of her Birth Plan. With the unfamiliarity and stress of labor, you might welcome an experienced, calm advocate who can remain with you through the birth.

If you use the above suggestions, not only will you be a more effective birth partner, but you will make your own role easier and more personally rewarding.

5

Strategies for Difficult Labors

*L*abor, even when perfectly normal, rarely follows a predictable "textbook" pattern. Variations within a range of normal are to be expected. The emotional reactions of women in labor vary, depending on the type of labor pattern they experience. For example, if prelabor or early labor drags on for a long time, the mother may be overcome with exhaustion, worry, or a loss of confidence. If, instead, labor starts suddenly with long, painful contractions that threaten to overwhelm the mother, her pain and panic are your main concerns. Women and their birth partners work best with labor when they are open and flexible, and when they are confident that they can and will (with the help of their caregivers) handle whatever comes their way.

This chapter covers situations that require special strategies and special understanding. These situations add stress and require more of the two of you—more resourcefulness, more effort, more decision making, more patience, more active coaching, and

133

more reliance on a doula or the caregiver and on medical or surgical interventions. The special situations covered here are

> The Take-Charge Routine (for Labor's Toughest Moments)
> On-the-Spot Coaching (When You Have Had No Childbirth Classes)
> The Slow-to-Start Labor
> The Very Rapid Labor
> The Emergency Delivery
> When Labor Must Start (Labor-Stimulating Measures)
> Backache During Labor
> When the Mother Must Labor in Bed
> A Breech Baby
> A Previous Disappointing Birth Experience
> Incompatibility with the Nurse or Caregiver

The Take-Charge Routine

Reserve this routine for any time during labor when the mother reacts in any of these ways:

- She hits an emotional low.
- She is in despair, weeps, or cries out.
- She wants to give up or feels she cannot go on.
- She is very tense and cannot relax.
- She is in a great deal of pain.
- She is unable to maintain a rhythmic ritual.

The Take-Charge Routine is exactly that. You move in close and do all you can to help the mother until she regains her inner strength. Usually her despair is brief; with your help she can pass through it and her spirits will rise. Use whatever parts of this routine seem appropriate:

- *Remain calm.* Your touch should be firm and confident, not anxious and tense. Your voice should remain calm and encouraging. Your facial expression should reflect confidence and optimism.
- *Stay close.* Face her or stay right by her side, your face near hers.
- *Anchor her.* Hold her shoulders or her head in your hands— gently, confidently, firmly—or hold her tightly in your arms.

- *Make eye contact.* Tell her to open her eyes and look at you. Say it loudly enough for her to hear you—but calmly and kindly.
- *Change the ritual she has been using during contractions.* Suggest a different position. Try changing the breathing pattern. Pace her breathing or moaning with your hand or voice.
- *Encourage her every breath.* Say "Breathe with me. . . . BREATHE WITH ME. . . . That's the way, . . . just like that. . . . Good. . . . Keep your rhythm. . . . STAY WITH IT. . . just like that. . . . LOOK AT ME. . . . Keep your rhythm. . . . Good for you. . . . It's going away. . . . Good. . . . Good. . . . Now just rest, that was so good." You can whisper these words or say them in a calm, rhythmic, and encouraging tone of voice. Sometimes you have to raise your voice to get her attention, but do not shout. And try to keep your tone calm and confident.
- *Talk to her between contractions.* Ask her if what you are doing is helping. Make suggestions: for example, "With the next one, let me help you more. I want you to look at me the moment it starts. We will breathe together so it won't get ahead of us. Okay? Good. You're doing so well. We're really moving now."
- *Repeat yourself.* She may not be able to continue doing what you tell her for more than a few seconds, but that's fine. Do not conclude that what you did did not help at all. Say the same things again and again, and help her continue.

What if she says she can't or won't go on? Here are some guidelines:

- *Don't give up on her.* This is a difficult time for her. You cannot help her if you decide she cannot handle it. Acknowledge to her and to yourself that it is difficult, but remind yourselves that it is not impossible.
- *Ask for help and reassurance.* The nurse, caregiver, or another support person can help a lot: measuring dilation, giving you advice, doing some of the coaching, trying something new, even reassuring you that the mother is okay and that this is normal.
- *Remind the mother of her baby.* It may seem surprising, but women can get so caught up in labor that they do not think

THE TAKE-CHARGE ROUTINE

much about their baby. It may help her to remember why she is going through all this.

What about pain medications? Do you call for them or not? It depends on

- The mother's prior wishes: Did she want an unmedicated birth? How strongly did she feel about it? (See the "Pain Medications Preference Scale," page 249.) Sometimes women who ask for pain medications are really saying, "I need more help."
- Her rate of progress and how far she still has to go. A couple of centimeters of progress should be very encouraging. A complete lack of progress is very discouraging.
- How well she responds to your more active coaching.
- Whether she is asking for medications herself, rather than agreeing to someone's suggestion, and how easily she can be talked out of them.

These considerations can help you decide what to do. It is sometimes difficult to balance present wishes against prior wishes. Try to stick with what the mother wanted before labor regarding the use of medication. But if she insists on changing the plan, respect her wishes. Numerous women have said, "I never could have done it without my partner. If it hadn't been for him [or her], I would have given up." By using the Take-Charge Routine, you can indeed get the mother through those desperate moments when she feels she cannot go on; you can truly ease her burden by helping her with every breath.

On-the-Spot Coaching (When You Have Had No Childbirth Classes)

If the due date nears and you have taken no childbirth classes, or if you took only a very short, "crash" course, you should consider hiring a doula to help you comfort the mother and guide the two of you through labor. But what if you have no doula, and labor starts early? What if you and the mother have had no time to work together to learn the pain-relief techniques described in chapter 4? Here are some suggestions: (1) Don't try to learn everything at once while the mother is in labor; (2) use some simple breathing patterns and a few on-the-spot comfort measures; (3) be sure to tell the staff that you and the mother have had no classes. Ask them to show you what to do.

Breathing Patterns

Once the contractions become uncomfortable, the mother can use patterned breathing during each one. You can breathe the pattern with her (be sure you do not have bad breath), verbally pace her through it, or conduct her breathing with rhythmic hand signals. Learn the *slow breathing* to use in early labor and *light breathing* (both page 107) to use later, if she needs it. Both patterns are simple and quick to learn. Have her practice between contractions.

With each out-breath, encourage the mother to release tension. As she breathes out you might say, "Let go here," and touch her shoulder, brow, or whatever part of her body is tense.

On-the-Spot Comfort Measures

Here are other on-the-spot comfort measures to try:

Movement and position changes (page 111)
Counterpressure (page 127)
Bath or shower (page 115)
Heat or cold (page 123)
Touch or massage (page 125)
Relaxation (page 103)
Attention-focusing (page 104)
The Take-Charge Routine (page 134)

Most of these measures can be used fairly well without much preparation. In fact, you can read about them while the mother is in labor and apply them immediately.

The Slow-to-Start Labor

Sometimes it takes hours or days of contractions before the cervix finally lets go and begins to dilate. We don't know exactly why this happens to some women and not to others, but the following conditions seem to predispose a woman to a slow-to-start labor:

- The mother's cervix is long (or thick), firm, and posterior when contractions begin (see "Labor Progresses in Six Ways," page 50).
- Her cervix is scarred from previous surgery or injury. A scarred cervix may resist thinning, and so may require more time and more intense contractions to overcome this resistance. Once thinning has occurred, labor usually progresses normally.
- Her uterus is contracting in an uncoordinated fashion, so that the contractions do not open the cervix. The reason for this is not understood.
- The baby is high in the mother's pelvis, because of the position of the head (see page 52). This is not necessarily a problem if the mother has previously given birth. In fact, if a woman has had a child before, the baby usually does not drop into the pelvis until after labor is well underway.
- The mother is very anxious and tense about the labor or the baby. Increased production of stress hormones can interfere with labor.
- Other unknown conditions may play a role.

No one can predict the course of the mother's labor, even if some of these conditions exist. Most slow-to-start labors eventually hit their stride and proceed normally after the initial long prelabor period. Some slow-to-start labors, however, are part of a generally prolonged labor, in which all phases proceed, but at a very slow pace. This type of labor presents a serious challenge to the mother and to her birth partner. You cannot know in advance just when her labor will speed up—only time will tell. Your role as birth partner will be to maintain the mother's morale and help her pace herself mentally and physically to accept slow progress.

Strategies for a Slow-to-Start Labor

If the mother's long prelabor is tiring and discouraging, though not necessarily painful, the following measures will help:

- Do not become discouraged yourself. Be patient and confident. This labor will *not* go on forever, and your positive attitude will help the mother keep her spirits up.
- If she is worried, remind her that *a long prelabor does not mean that anything is wrong* with her or the baby. Her cervix simply needs more time before it thins and begins opening. The two of you need to find ways to wait without worrying.
- Call her friends, family, caregiver, or childbirth educator for encouragement and morale boosting. Do not call anyone who is going to make you worry more.
- Try not to become preoccupied with the labor or to overreact to every contraction. This only makes it seem longer.
- Encourage the mother to eat and drink high-carbohydrate, easily digested foods (for example, toast with jam, cereals, pancakes, pasta, fruit juice, tea with sugar or honey, sorbet or gelatin desserts).

Additionally, you can help her pass the time by rotating among distracting, restful, and labor-stimulating activities. Here are some suggestions:

1. Try *distracting activities* during the day. Encourage the mother to get out of the house. If she is willing, she can visit friends; go for a walk; go to work (let her decide whether she can); go to a movie, the shopping mall, or a restaurant (you can hope you'll have to leave before you're done!). You'll find that when she is out of the house she will try to minimize the contractions. This is easier for her to do when she is among other people than when she's alone at home.

At home you can try these distracting activities: watch TV programs or videos that *she* likes; dance; play some favorite music; clean; straighten up; pay bills; play games; start a time-consuming project, such as baking bread or painting a crib (she will almost hope that labor doesn't start until the project is finished!); fix meals for after the baby is born; have friends over, especially to relieve you if you are tired.

2. Help her rest or sleep at night, or nap during the day, if possible. If she is tired but cannot sleep, try the following:

- If a long prelabor has fatigued and discouraged her, suggest a bath. Fill the tub with warm (not hot) water; provide an inflatable bathtub pillow or folded towels for a headrest. She should plan to stay in the tub for a long time; you may have to add hot water from time to time. Rest and sleep come more easily in a warm bath. Keep an eye on her; make sure she doesn't slip down so her head goes under the water. Remember that a bath tends to slow contractions in early labor, and should be used then only when a woman needs a rest.

- If no bath is available, encourage the mother to try a long shower. You might need to turn up the water heater.
- Play some soothing music.
- Give her a soothing massage.
- Give her a relaxing beverage (warm milk, herbal tea).
- Use relaxation techniques and slow breathing during contractions.

3. Try labor-stimulating measures for periods of one or two hours at a time to initiate stronger, more frequent contractions. Follow the guidelines in "When Labor Must Start," page 147, noting the precautions for these procedures.

4. If the mother is not only sleepless, but is also in pain, long baths, relaxation, massage, and slow patterned breathing will help. See "Self-Help Comfort Measures," page 102, for ideas.

5. Especially if she has back pain and irregular contractions, the open knee-chest position (see page 113) may help; have her keep this position on a bed for 30 to 45 minutes, using pillows for support. In an OP position (see page 44) this may help to back the baby's head out of the pelvis, giving it a chance to reposition before coming down again. Contractions may even stop for a while. Or try abdominal lifting (see page 155) during rather than between contractions. This may realign the baby more favorably with her pelvis and reduce some of her pain.

If these strategies are not enough to get her through a long prelabor, her caregiver may give her morphine or another drug (see page 238).

If you are worried that the mother won't have the stamina to cope with "real" labor after this prolonged prelabor, remind yourself—and her—that she is well equipped at this time in her life to cope with a long period without sleep. Women's energy levels increase before labor as their bodies gear up for the physical demands ahead. The mother may handle it better than you do! The nesting urge is evidence of this extraordinary bodily adjustment. Try to have confidence that, although it may be difficult, the odds are excellent that she will have the energy it takes to handle the later phases of labor.

The Very Rapid Labor

Some women have labors that start with hard, frequent, painful contractions and are over in a matter of a few hours. It seems the mother barely has time to adjust to being in labor before the baby is born. Or, sometimes only the first (dilation) stage is rapid: the cervix dilates so quickly that the mother can't catch up mentally; but then, in the second (birthing) stage, the uterus takes a long rest. If that happens, the mother has to cope with the difficulties of both fast and slow labors. It is impossible to predict which women will labor in these ways, but a rapid labor seems to be more likely if

- The mother has had a rapid or quicker-than-average (less than 10 hours) labor before. A second or third labor tends to be faster than the first.
- Her cervix is very soft, thin, and already partially dilated before labor begins, and the baby is low in the mother's pelvis in a favorable position.

Few women or their birth partners are prepared for a rapid labor, especially after reading and learning about typical labor patterns and prolonged prelabors. If the mother's labor starts rapidly, she will be caught off guard: she was expecting the early contractions to be gentle, short, and far apart; but her labor begins instead with contractions that are long, painful, and close together—almost like the contractions of the transition phase.

How Is the Mother Likely to React?

You can expect the following reactions from the mother if her labor begins rapidly:

- *Shock and disbelief.* She may not be able to respond constructively. She may not realize that this is real labor.

- *Fear or panic.* She may think that something is terribly wrong—that she or the baby is in danger. Or, she may be frightened that she cannot reach you, her caregiver, or anyone else for help, or that she cannot get to the hospital in time.
- *Loss of confidence.* If the mother thinks these are the "easy" contractions of early labor, she may lose all confidence that she can cope with labor once it progresses.
- *Dependence on you.* She may barely be able to change positions between contractions, let alone get ready to go to the hospital. She may need your constant help to cope with the contractions.

How Should You React?

- Believe what you see. If the mother is shaky, in pain, having strong, fast contractions, don't assume she is overreacting to early labor. Assume she is having a hard labor and move right into a leadership role in helping her cope.
- Use the "Take-Charge Routine" (page 134) if she has trouble with the contractions.
- Don't lose faith in her or criticize her. Don't conclude she has less fortitude than you had thought. Her response truly reflects how hard this labor is.
- Call the caregiver, go to the hospital, or both. Drive carefully, but don't waste time.

The Emergency Delivery

What if it is too late to get to the hospital? What if you and the mother are on your own—in your car or at home? How will you know if it's too late to go to the hospital? What if the baby is coming? If this is a planned home birth, what if the midwife has not arrived? You will know that it is too late to go to the hospital if (1) the mother says she can feel the baby coming out; (2) you can see the baby's head at her vaginal opening; or (3) she is pushing and grunting forcibly and cannot stop. If all of this happens at home, stay there and call 911 for an emergency vehicle with a paramedical team. Also try to call the hospital.

If all this happens in the car, pull over to the side of the road, put on your flasher lights, and tend to the mother's needs. If the weather is cold, leave the motor running and the heater on—you don't want the baby to get chilled once he is born. (Be sure the emergency brake is on!)

Basic Rules for an Emergency Delivery

Before the birth, this is what you do:

- Believe the mother if she says the baby is coming.
- Remain calm (at least try to act calm!).
- Get help: from paramedics (call 911), friends or neighbors, even children.
- Turn up the heat in the car or at home.
- Gather blankets, towels, or warm clothing to wrap the baby in.
- Find newspapers, a bowl, paper towels, or a plastic bag to hold the placenta.
- Reassure the mother. Point out that when labor happens this fast, it's because there's *nothing* holding it up; in fact, everything is working too well.
- Help the mother breathe through her contractions. She SHOULD NOT PUSH. Help her pant or blow lightly with her chin up when her body starts to push. This is to slow the delivery.
- Help the mother lie down on her side or recline in a semi-sitting position if possible; this is preferable to squatting or standing. Lying down may slow the delivery slightly, and it ensures that the baby will have a safe place to land as he comes out.
- Get ready to catch the baby. Have something ready to dry and cover the baby immediately (towels, blanket, your shirt or jacket).
- Make sure the baby lands in a soft place (on the bed or the seat of the car), and does not drop. Babies come out fast and are very wet and slippery, so you may not be able to catch him. If the woman is standing or squatting, or if there is no soft place for the baby to land, place your body so that the baby will land on you if you don't catch him.
- Wash your hands thoroughly, if possible, but this is not so

important that you should leave the mother if she needs you badly or if the baby is coming out.

As the baby comes out, this is what you do:

- Help the mother to pant, not push.
- Wipe the baby's face and head when it emerges. If the membranes of the bag of waters cover the baby's face (which is very unlikely), tear them with your fingernail or remove them by pulling at them with a towel so the baby can breathe. When the baby's head is out, it will turn toward one side, and then the shoulders and body will probably be born with the next contraction.
- Catch the baby.
- Wipe the baby off and quickly place him naked on his side or stomach on his mother's naked abdomen. Skin-to-skin contact is the best way to keep him warm. Cover him (including his head but not his face) with a blanket, towel, or clothing. It is critical to keep the baby dry and warm. You'll want to be able to see his face to monitor his condition.
- Check the baby's breathing. Babies normally begin breathing or crying within seconds after birth. Wipe away any mucus, blood, or vernix (a white, creamy substance that may be found all over the baby) from his nostrils or mouth.
- Rub the baby's head, back, or chest briskly or slap the soles of his feet if he doesn't begin breathing right away. He might sputter and choke out some mucus or fluid from his airway.
- Don't lay the baby on his back; that position would make it harder for him to get rid of any fluids that might be in his nose, mouth, or chest. Place the baby on his side or, preferably, on his stomach with his head lower than his body. This "safety position" is the best to promote breathing. Be sure the baby's face is clear for breathing and not pressed into the mother's body.

The Cord and the Placenta. Don't worry about the cord at all. You do not need to cut it or tie it. Changes within the cord cause compression of the blood vessels and stop blood flow through the cord within a few minutes after the birth.

The placenta will probably be born within 30 minutes after the baby is born. If it seems slow in coming, have the mother stand or squat. Do not pull on the cord—just let it come. Catch the placenta in a bowl, a towel, a blanket, or in a piece of clothing. Place it near the baby's body. It will be bloody and messy, but it is otherwise not a problem.

Care of the Mother. You can expect some bleeding from the mother's vagina, but if it looks like more than two cups of blood, she may be losing too much. Do the following, whether the mother is bleeding excessively or not:

- Place the baby at the mother's breast as soon as possible after delivery (when you know he is breathing and even before the placenta comes, if the cord is long enough to allow it). The baby's suckling or just nuzzling at the breast helps contract the uterus and slow down any bleeding.
- Feel the mother's abdomen for her uterus by pressing into the area below her navel. It should feel hard and firm, like a large grapefruit. If you cannot feel the uterus, it is because it is too relaxed. You should get it to contract tightly because a *relaxed uterus bleeds too much*. (See "When the Mother Bleeds Excessively," page 146.)

Once both mother and baby appear to be all right, you should get them to the hospital for a thorough checkup. The mother might need stitches; the baby will need to have his cord cared for and to have a physical exam. Other procedures may be appropriate as well.

Your caregiver (especially if you had originally planned a home birth) or the paramedical team will probably have arrived by this time. You will be very relieved. Some day, this will make a great story to tell at parties and baby showers!

First Aid for Emergencies in Childbirth

What if the emergency birth doesn't go so normally? You should know a little about this possibility, just in case a complication arises.

The two major complications of emergency deliveries are these: the mother bleeds excessively or the baby does not begin to breathe. These complications, though rare, can present real dangers. The following discussion explains what to do if they happen. Of course, if you have had time to call an ambulance, you will very likely have medical help soon; but you must know what to do until help arrives.

When the Mother Bleeds Excessively. The mother will have some bleeding, but if it looks as if she is losing more than two cups of blood, or if she gets weak and pale and her skin feels clammy, she may be losing too much. This could happen because of bleeding from her uterus, before or after the placenta comes out, or because of bleeding from open wounds in the vagina or perineum (the area between the vagina and the anus) caused by the rapid birth. Following are some guidelines for preventing excessive bleeding.

If the placenta is out, get the uterus to contract in these ways:

1. *Stimulate the mother's nipples.* Having the baby suckle at the breast is most effective; try this first. If the baby is not ready to suckle, try rolling the nipples between your fingers (or have the mother do it herself). Roll both nipples at the same time or roll one while the baby suckles at the other.

2. *Massage the top of her uterus* (the fundus) in her lower abdomen with one or both hands vigorously until the uterus contracts. This is painful to the mother, but do not stop until the uterus hardens. It will feel like a grapefruit, in size and consistency, when it has contracted.

If the placenta has not come out within 30 minutes, try stimulating the mother's nipples and help her to kneel, squat, or stand. You must get her to the hospital to have the placenta removed if these measures are not immediately successful. *Do not pull on the cord.*

It is very hard to tell if the source of excessive bleeding is a tear or laceration (cut) in the vagina or perineum. But if you can see that there is a tear or laceration, place ice wrapped in a wet cloth or towel in the vagina and apply firm pressure. Go to the hospital.

If the mother becomes weak, pale, and shaky, and her skin becomes clammy, then her blood pressure has fallen too low. Lay her down with her head level with or lower than the rest of her body.

When the Baby Does Not Begin to Breathe. If the baby does not begin to breathe within 2 minutes after you have wiped fluids away from her nose and mouth, you need to use infant CPR (cardiopulmonary resuscitation):

1. Rub the baby's trunk and head briskly.
2. Check the baby's mouth and remove any blobs of mucus you find.
3. Lay the baby on her back, and gently bend her head back.
4. Place your mouth over both the baby's nose and mouth, and, with your hand on her chest, blow gently until her chest rises a little. Repeat this every 3 seconds until the baby breathes on her own or until help arrives. *Don't blow hard:* a baby's lungs are tiny. You need to blow only enough to make the baby's chest rise.
5. Get to the hospital as soon as possible.

When the midwife or paramedical team arrives or you get to the hospital, the emergency personnel will have drugs to contract the uterus, intravenous fluids, oxygen and resuscitation equipment to help the baby breathe, and (in the hospital) everything they need to remove a retained placenta. Most hospitals are ready for immediate action.

You will probably feel lost in the shuffle. Try to stay with the mother or the baby, but recognize that in an obstetric emergency, immediate action is the primary concern and you must not impede it in any way. In a true emergency, there may be no time until afterwards for explanations or answers to your questions.

When Labor Must Start (Labor-Stimulating Measures)

Under some circumstances, the caregiver decides that delaying or awaiting the baby's birth for much longer carries unacceptable risks to mother or baby. Then, the caregiver must consider artificially inducing labor (starting labor with drugs or by breaking the bag of waters). The caregiver will consider inducing labor under the following circumstances:

• The mother has an illness such as diabetes, heart disease, lung disease, or high blood pressure.

FIRST AID FOR EMERGENCIES IN CHILDBIRTH

- There is no herpes lesion in a woman who has been plagued by frequent outbreaks of herpes, and her due date is near.
- The pregnancy has lasted 42 weeks or more.
- The bag of waters has been broken for a prolonged period.
- The fetus has grown slowly and is too small (because of poor functioning of the placenta).
- The fetus seems overly stressed in the uterus.

Under other circumstances, such as a prolonged prelabor or a slowdown in active labor, the caregiver, the mother, or both may want to speed up or strengthen (augment) the contractions by breaking the bag of waters or using intravenous oxytocin.

The mother may be able to start labor herself with the following measures. If she is successful, she can avoid a medical induction of labor, which carries some risk and is invasive. (See "Induction and Augmentation of Labor," page 189.) If she is not successful, she may end up with an induction anyway.

Before using these techniques to stimulate labor, be sure the mother discusses them with her caregiver. She should ask the caregiver whether there is any reason that she should not try to stimulate contractions, and, if not, how to do it.

Nipple Stimulation

Stimulating the mother's nipples causes the release of oxytocin, a hormone that contracts the uterus. Taking advantage of this physiological connection between breast and uterus may start labor or at least cause some contractions. Nipple stimulation probably will not work, however, in a woman who is currently breastfeeding a toddler; her body has adapted to increased levels of oxytocin.

Methods of Nipple Stimulation. The following measures might need to be repeated after a few hours or after half a day. Either you or the mother can stimulate the nipples in the following ways:

- Lightly stroke, roll, or brush one or both nipples with the fingertips. Often, within a few minutes the mother will have stronger contractions. You or she may need to continue this stimulation for hours to keep the contractions coming.
- Massage the breasts gently with warm, moist towels for an

hour at a time, three times a day.

- Caress, lick, or suck the mother's nipples, or roll them between your fingers. Try this for as long as the mother finds it effective and pleasant, or until her contractions become strong.
- Use a gentle, but powerful, institutional-quality electric breast pump (available in hospitals). A nurse can show her what to do. Manual or battery-operated breast pumps are less likely to be useful.
- Nurse a borrowed baby. Suckling a three- to twelve-week-old baby seems to be the most effective form of nipple stimulation. At this age babies are usually efficient nursers but are not too fussy to suckle at the breast of someone besides their mother. The woman's midwife or childbirth educator may be able to help her find the right baby. The baby should not have an oral thrush infection, which could be spread to the mother's nipples.

    If the woman is ill, she should not try this—the baby could catch her illness.

    The baby needs to be awake and not very hungry. A sleepy baby will not suck, and a hungry baby gets frustrated by the lack of milk. The baby's fussy period is a good time, because the baby often wants simply to suck.

    Before nursing a borrowed baby, the woman should wash her breasts and hands. Because her waters may break, she should sit on a waterproof pad. She should try to suckle the baby for at least 10 minutes on each side.

If the mother is uncomfortable with the idea of nursing someone else's baby, try the other methods of nipple stimulation and of bringing on labor (see pages 147 to 149).

Precautions When Using Nipple Stimulation. Many caregivers are very comfortable with their clients' use of nipple stimulation to bring on labor, but others are wary, because stimulating the nipples occasionally causes excessively long or strong contractions. These caregivers worry that strong contractions may stress the fetus, especially if the mother is at high risk for complications. Before advising nipple stimulation, the caregiver may want to check the fetal response to such stimulation by having the mother first try it during electronic fetal monitoring.

If the contractions are not too long or intense and the baby tolerates them well, then the caregiver may feel it will be safe to continue nipple stimulation at home. It is wise to also take the following precautions to help avoid excessively strong or long contractions:

1. Time the length and assess the intensity of all contractions resulting from nipple stimulation.

2. Begin with "low-dose," intermittent stimulation and work up as needed. At first, stimulate one nipple until the mother has a contraction; then stop until the contraction is over. Repeat. Try this for four to six contractions.

3. If stimulating only one nipple does not cause any contractions in a reasonable length of time, or if the contractions the mother is already having do not increase in frequency, length, or strength, try stimulating both breasts intermittently, then, if necessary, both breasts continuously. Having the mother nurse a baby is probably the most effective form of stimulation.

4. Stop altogether if the "low-dose" stimulation results in contractions that are painful or long (over 60 seconds).

Walking

Although more effective in speeding a slow labor, walking may also help to get labor started. You might try taking the mother for a fairly brisk walk, but don't go too far away from home or the labor room.

Acupressure

Certain acupressure (*shiatsu*) points can be activated to stimulate contractions. Although acupressure is little understood in Western cultures, it is widely practiced in the Far East for health purposes. One point, Spleen 6, is considered a powerful point; when pressure is applied there, it can induce contractions of the uterus. This point should not be pressed before the mother's due date.

Use acupressure in the following way to stimulate contractions:

1. Locate Spleen 6, about four finger breadths (hers, not yours) above her inner ankle on the shinbone. This is a very tender spot.

2. Press the Spleen 6 point firmly with the tip of your thumb, on the bone and toward the front of her leg. See the illustration and further discussion of Spleen 6 on page 125.

3. Apply the pressure three times for 10 to 60 seconds at a time, resting for 10 to 60 seconds in between.

4. Repeat the cycle every few minutes if the pressure seems to be causing contractions.

Sexual Stimulation

Intercourse with orgasm is the most effective form of sexual stimulation in starting labor. Orgasm causes the release of oxytocin and contractions of the uterus, and may also cause the release of other hormone-like substances (prostaglandins), which soften the cervix. Semen is a rich source of postaglandins, too. Clitoral stimulation, even without orgasm or intercourse, may also be somewhat effective in bringing on contractions.

If you choose these methods of stimulation, make them as pleasant as possible. Try to forget your goal of starting labor and free yourselves to enjoy the sexual experience.

There are a few precautions to follow when using these methods:

1. You may use intercourse, manual stimulation of the clitoris, and oral sexual stimulation as long as the mother's bag of waters is intact, but avoid placing anything within the vagina if the membranes have ruptured, because doing so would increase the risk of infection.

2. Never blow into the vagina during pregnancy.

3. Modify or avoid these methods if either of you has any sores that could spread or if the mother has an uncomfortable vaginal condition.

Bowel Stimulation

The mother may be able to start labor by taking castor oil to stimulate and empty her bowels. A laxative, castor oil may cause powerful contractions of the bowels, and diarrhea. The oil has been used to induce labor for years and years, with some success. Some experts believe this method increases the mother's level of prostaglandins, which are produced when the bowels contract. The prostaglandins cause the cervix to soften and thin.

Be sure the mother checks with her caregiver before using castor oil. If the caregiver approves, follow these guidelines:

1. Give the mother 4 tablespoons (2 ounces) of unflavored castor oil to start. Castor oil is more palatable if you mix it with an equal amount of orange juice and a teaspoon of baking soda; stir the mixture fast. She should drink it quickly. Or make the oil palatable by mixing it with scrambled eggs.

2. One-half hour later, the mother may take 2 tablespoons more oil in the same way.

3. After another half-hour she may take another 2 tablespoons. The mother should take no more than three doses, totaling 4 ounces.

Do not expect contractions immediately. When the method works, contractions pick up within half a day. But sometimes castor oil may only improve the readiness of the cervix to dilate, and labor is started the next day through nipple stimulation or another method.

Enemas, previously used for starting labor, have been found ineffective for this purpose, even though they do help empty the bowels.

Teas and Tinctures

Some midwives and physicians use certain herbal teas or tinctures (for example, blue or black cohosh tea) to bring on or speed up contractions. Use these teas or tinctures only under the guidance of the mother's caregiver, as dosage and strength should be individualized, and potential side effects explained.

Backache During Labor

One woman in three or four feels intense backache during labor contractions. Relaxation and breathing are usually not enough to cope with the pain.

Back labor is usually the result of the baby's position. Most often, the baby is head down, facing forward in the mother's body, with the back of the head pressing against the mother's low spine. This is called the OP (occiput posterior) position and it causes intense pain in the low spine (see page 44). Other malpositions, such as a tilted head and a raised chin, may also cause back pain.

Most OP babies rotate spontaneously during labor, turning their heads until the back of the head is pointing toward the mother's front (in the OA, or occiput anterior, position). This rotation can take place at any time during labor—early or late. Other malpositions also resolve in time. There is often a delay in dilation in the active phase while the baby's head rotates. Once the baby has rotated, the back pain usually subsides, and labor progress resumes.

Occasionally, the baby does not rotate by herself, with the following possible consequences: (1) labor may be very slow if the baby is also large; (2) the baby may be born facing forward ("sunny-side up"), though such a birth is rare; (3) the caregiver may assist the delivery with forceps or a vacuum extractor after the cervix is fully dilated (see page 199); (4) a cesarean delivery may be the solution if vaginal birth appears too difficult.

You can help the mother deal with backache in labor by (1) encouraging the baby to rotate and (2) using specific comfort measures to relieve the mother's back pain.

Encourage the Baby to Rotate

Try to find out the position of the baby. The mother may be able to figure out its position by locating the places she feels most of the baby's small movements, like kicking and punching: the baby's hand and foot movements are probably directly opposite where its back is. The nurse or caregiver can usually tell where it is by palpating the mother's abdomen and feeling parts of the baby. If the back of the baby's head is pressing against the mother's back, the mother will feel most of the baby's small movements in the front of her abdomen, to the left or right side of center.

Once you know that the baby is in an OP position, help the mother to use different body positions, pelvic rocking, and abdominal stroking to encourage the baby to turn. Even if you are not sure that the baby is OP, if the mother has backache during her contractions, try these measures. They tend to relieve discomfort, and they will *not* turn an OA baby into an OP position.

Positions and Movements to Try in Early Labor. The following positions and movements encourage a baby in OP position to rotate to OA, while relieving backache. With some of them (abdominal stroking, the lunge, sidelying, and lying semi-prone), it helps to know whether the baby is right occiput posterior (ROP), with the back of the baby's head pointing toward the right side of the mother's back, or left occiput posterior (LOP), with the back of the baby's head pointing toward the left side of the mother's back (see the illustrations on page 44).

- *The open knee-chest position.* From her hands and knees, the mother lowers her head and chest down to the floor or bed. Be sure her buttocks are high in the air and her hips are open enough that her knees are further from her belly than her hips. She should remain in this position for 30 to 45 minutes, even though the back pain may subside immediately as soon as she gets into this position. Though the position is awkward, try to help her maintain it by encouraging her to lean on you or by supporting her shoulders (see pages 116 to 117).
- *Pelvic rocking.* While kneeling and leaning forward, the mother rocks her pelvis forward and back, or in a circle. This helps to ease the mother's backache and to dislodge the baby within her pelvis, encouraging rotation whether the baby is ROP or LOP (see page 20).
- *Abdominal stroking.* While the mother is on hands and knees, reach beneath her abdomen and firmly stroke repeat-

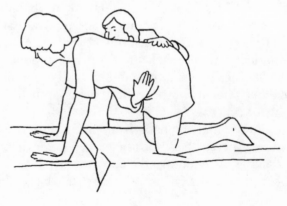

edly across her abdomen in the direction the baby should rotate—from the side of her body where the baby's back is to the other side. If the caregiver says the baby is ROP, stroke from right to left; if the baby is LOP, stroke from left to right. The stroking should feel good. It is usually better to do it between, not during, contractions. Don't do it if it is uncomfortable or if you do not know whether the baby is ROP or LOP.

- *Abdominal lifting.* While standing, the mother interlocks her fingers and places them against her pubic bone. During contractions, she lifts her abdomen up and slightly in, while bending her knees. This often relieves back pain while improving the position of the baby in the pelvis. You may be able to help her by standing behind her and lifting her abdomen.

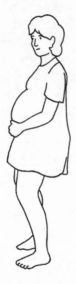

She can alternate these measures with restful positions.

Positions and Movements to Try in Active Labor. If she still has backache or if her labor has begun to slow down, she should continue pelvic rocking or abdominal lifting, but not the open knee-chest position or abdominal stroking. Also try these:

- *Slow dancing.* You embrace the mother as you stand face to face, and the two of you sway from side to side. This pleasant alternative to walking helps to relieve backache and to rotate the baby, even if you do not know whether he's ROP or LOP (see page 116).

- *The lunge.* Have the mother stand beside a chair, with one foot on the chair seat and her raised knee and foot pointing the side. Make sure the chair will not slide. Without bending at her waist, she slowly "lunges," or leans sideways, toward the chair. She should feel a stretch on the insides of both her thighs. She stays in the position for a slow count of 5, then returns to upright (see page 116).

  The mother can lunge either during or between contractions. If you know the baby's position, have her lunge toward the side where the baby's back is. If you do not know the baby's position, have her try lunging in each direction, and stick with the direction that is the most comfortable. Help the mother with her balance, and keep the chair from sliding.

- *Sidelying.* The mother lies on her side with both hips and knees flexed, and a pillow between her knees. If the baby is LOP, she lies on her left side; if ROP, on her right side; if you are not sure of the baby's position, have her turn from one side to the other every 20 to 30 minutes.

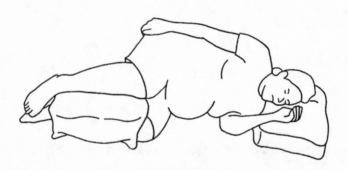

- *Lying semiprone.* If the baby's back is on her left side (LOP), the mother lies on her right side with her lower arm behind her and her lower leg out straight. She flexes her upper hip and knee, rests her knee on a doubled-up pillow and rolls toward her front. If the baby's back is on her right side, she lies the same way on her left side. If you are not sure of the baby's position, have the mother change sides every 20 to 30 minutes.

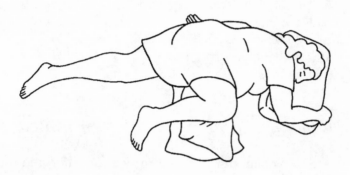

- *Kneeling and leaning forward.* The mother rests her upper body on a chair or a birth ball (see page 117). Some birthing beds can be adjusted to support this position.
- *Standing and walking.* These take advantage of gravity in encouraging the descent of the baby. In addition, the alignment of the baby within the pelvis is thought to be most favorable when the mother is upright. Also, walking allows some movement within the pelvic joints, which may encourage the baby's rotation.

BACKACHE DURING LABOR

Comfort Measures for Backache

Along with the measures already suggested for turning the baby, there are some comfort measures that are particularly useful in reducing back pain. These comfort measures, described in chapter 4, include the following:

Counterpressure (page 127)
Touch and Massage (page 125)
Heat and Cold (page 123)
The Double Hip Squeeze (page 126)
The Knee Press (page 126)
Rolling Pressure Over the Low Back (page 129)
Baths and Showers (page 115)
Transcutaneous Electrical Nerve Stimulation (TENS, page 123)

When the Mother Must Labor in Bed

Sometimes a woman must remain in bed for labor and birth. These are the most common reasons:

- The mother has high blood pressure. A woman's blood pressure tends to lower when she lies on her left side.
- The mother has used pain medications. If a woman is sleepy or groggy, or if part of her body is numb, she is safest staying in bed.
- The mother needs to use equipment that attaches her to machines. Intravenous fluids, electric infusion pumps (for pitocin drip), electronic fetal monitors, catheters, and others all tend to make it difficult or impossible for the woman to move out of bed.
- It is the hospital's custom. Unfortunately, in many hospitals women are routinely discouraged from leaving their beds. There is no medical reason for such a practice.

Being restricted to bed may present no particular problems for the mother, especially if it does not add to her pain, or if she had not expected to do anything else. Many women, however, find lying down to be most uncomfortable. Some women become very restless and are unable to stay down. If they had planned to use movement and positioning for comfort or to help their labors progress, they will be disappointed and will want to change their caregiver's orders.

Sometimes restricting a woman to bed slows her labor and increases the pain from contractions. She is also prevented from doing many of the things that speed labor and increase her comfort.

Here are some things you should do if the mother is confined to bed:

1. Find out why. You and she may be able to persuade her caregiver to change the orders if there is no compelling medical reason for the mother to remain in bed. If bed rest is medically necessary, you will both be better able to accept it and cooperate if you understand why.

2. Find out how strict the order is. The mother may be told not to leave the bed, or she may be told not to turn from her left side at all. She may be allowed up for short periods or to go to the bathroom. She may be able to take a bath, which could be as effective for lowering blood pressure as lying on her left side.

3. Ask about alternatives. The mother may be able to use a telemetry unit (see page 183) for electronic fetal monitoring and an IV pole on wheels. These would allow her to be out of bed and walking. Even if she is connected to many machines and containers, she may be able to stand or to sit in a rocker beside the bed.

4. Help her focus on the many pain-coping techniques and comfort measures she can use while in bed, without dwelling too much on what she cannot do. Try relaxation (page 102), patterned breathing (page 105), attention focusing (page 104), spontaneous rituals (page 100), counterpressure and other techniques for relieving back pain (page 127), massage and acupressure (pages 125 and 126), heat and cold (page 123), transcutaneous electrical nerve stimulation (TENS) (page 123), hypnosis (page 104), or the "Take-Charge Routine" (page 134).

Remaining in bed sometimes adds to the mother's stress, but, with your help, she can probably handle this challenge. The key is to understand and accept the reasons she must remain in bed, to focus on the techniques she can still use, and to make sure she has excellent labor support.

A Breech Baby

In late pregnancy, about 1 in 30 babies is in a breech presentation (with head up and buttocks or feet, or both, down at the mother's cervix). Many breech babies turn spontaneously to a head-down position, but fewer do so close to term than at 34 weeks or earlier. There are three types of breech presentation: the *frank* breech, with the buttocks down at the cervix; the *complete* breech, with the knees bent so that both buttocks and feet are down at the cervix; and the *footling* breech, with one or both feet down at the cervix.

A breech presentation presents more problems than most head-first presentations, particularly if the baby is premature or very large, and if the presentation is footling or complete breech. Briefly, the problems are as follows:

• The cord is more likely to prolapse (see page 209), especially in footling and complete breech presentations.
• Other difficulties are due mostly to the fact that the head is born last. Sometimes there is a delay in the birth of the head, because it is the largest part of the baby. Sometimes the baby inhales amniotic fluid and vaginal secretions, which can interfere with breathing after birth. Also, while still inside, the head can pinch the cord while the baby still depends on it for oxygen.

Because of these risks, most doctors today discourage vaginal delivery of a breech baby. In fact, obstetric training programs no longer teach doctors how to assist at breech births, so only a few have the skills. For these reasons, the following procedures may be recommended during late pregnancy, either to turn the baby to a head-down presentation, or to deliver the baby most safely.

Breech Tilt. At between 32 and 35 weeks' gestation, the mother may begin using the *breech tilt* position to encourage her baby to turn, as follows:

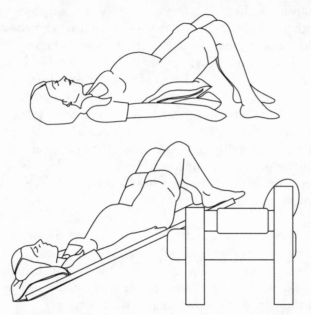

The breech tilt position, in two variants.

1. Three times a day, when her stomach is not full and her baby is active, she lies on the floor on her back with her knees bent and feet flat. She raises her hips 12 inches or more. You slide cushions beneath her hips to hold her in the tilted position. She is now lying with her head and shoulders on the floor and her hips and knees raised. The same position can be achieved by having her lie on an ironing board (or a board of similar length but wider) with one end propped on a couch.

2. She remains there for 10 to 15 minutes (less if she is uncomfortable).

3. As she consciously releases tension in her abdomen and trunk, she visualizes her baby's head pressing "down" against the top of the uterus, and the baby trying to get her head "up" again.

The position seems to encourage some babies to turn, but it may not work. Research studies have not found the breech tilt to be clearly more effective than doing nothing.

Music. If the mother has high blood pressure or cannot tolerate the breech tilt position, she should avoid it and concentrate on using music for the same purpose. Place stereo earphones low on the mother's abdomen and play rhythmic music at a volume that she finds comfortable. Some people believe babies particularly like Baroque music. The baby may try to move her head closer so she can hear the music better. The music can be used with or without the breech tilt position. This seems to work sometimes.

You might also try to get the baby to turn by lying down with your head in the mother's lap, facing her abdomen. Then call the baby (don't yell), and, at a normal voice level, tell her to come down so she can hear you better. Who knows—she just may flip so that she can better hear your voice, with which she is probably already familiar.

Breech Version. If the baby is still breech at 37 or 38 weeks' gestation, the mother and her caregiver may decide to try an *external version*, a procedure for turning a breech baby. Versions have been done over the years in many cultures. This is how they are done today in a medical setting:

1. The mother goes to the office or hospital. An ultrasound scan is performed to confirm the breech presentation and to assess the baby's size, the location of the placenta, the amount of amniotic fluid, and other conditions. An electronic fetal monitor is used to perform a nonstress test, an assessment of the baby's well-being (see page 180).

2. The mother is given an injection of terbutaline, which relaxes the uterus. She may also be given an epidural, to relax her abdominal muscles and prevent pain from the procedure.

3. She lies on her back and relaxes.

4. The doctor (midwives do not do these versions) rubs a lubricant on the mother's abdomen and, with the guidance of ultrasound, presses on her abdomen to lift the baby out of the pelvis and gradually turn the baby around so the head is down. If unsuccessful at first the doctor may try once or twice more, but usually not more than that.

5. The mother remains as relaxed as possible; your help with this makes a big difference, if she has had no epidural.

6. After the procedure, the mother undergoes another nonstress test (see page 181) to see that the baby has tolerated the procedure well.

7. The version procedure takes only 5 to 20 minutes, but if the mother has had an epidural she remains in the hospital until the medication wears off.

Although the version procedure has many built-in safeguards, most caregivers notify the labor and delivery floor that they are doing it, so if a serious problem should arise, such as prolapsed cord, fetal distress, or bleeding, a cesarean could be performed at once.

Versions are successful 60 to 70 percent of the time. Most of the women who undergo versions give birth vaginally to healthy babies.

When a version is not successful, a vaginal birth may be planned, if (1) the caregiver is experienced in vaginal breech births (and few are today), (2) the baby is no larger than average size, (3) the baby is in a frank breech presentation (only the buttocks are down), (4) the baby's chin is tucked down on his chest, and (5) the mother's pelvis appears to be of adequate size.

If all these conditions are not present, a cesarean birth is planned to assure the best possible outcome. The cesarean rate for breech presentation is very high in North America.

A Previous
Disappointing Birth Experience

Most women who have gone through labor have some doubts about whether they can "do it again." For those whose previous birth experiences were normal and satisfying, confidence and optimism tend to outweigh apprehension or doubt. But, for those who have had disappointing birth experiences such as a cesarean birth, a difficult, frightening, or traumatic birth, or a premature, sick, disabled, or stillborn baby, the memories of these past difficulties may keep coming back. As these women approach and anticipate the upcoming labor and birth, they may be haunted by various doubts and anxieties. For example, they may not feel confident about being able to cope with childbirth again; they may be anxious about their own safety, especially if their previous labor ended in a cesarean or in a difficult forceps or vacuum delivery; or they may be worried about the baby, especially if they had a baby who did not survive or who was very ill.

If the mother has had a previous difficult birth experience, she will benefit from special preparation for labor and special understanding and support during labor. The following suggestions should help you to help her:

- Look for books about giving birth after a previous cesarean, recovery from a traumatic birth experience, or pregnancy after the loss of a baby (see "Recommended Resources"). You both should read these books.
- Find a support group or a class that helps women and their partners prepare for labor after a previous disappointing birth experience. VBAC (vaginal birth after cesarean) classes, postpartum depression groups, and Pregnancy After Loss meetings are all available. These programs help the mother realize that she is not the only woman troubled by a previous difficult birth, and that she *can* cope. They also teach the birth partner how to be especially helpful during labor. Ask the caregiver or the hospital for the names of instructors or leaders of these classes and groups.
- Check the Internet for websites and e-mail groups that focus on difficult childbirths.
- Learn about labor and how to be a birth partner by reading this book and by taking childbirth classes, because the mother will need especially sensitive and capable labor support.
- Consider using the services of a doula. She can offer you and the mother her experienced perspective, steady encouragement, and specific help. She can also work with you and the staff as a go-between or advocate.

You should also anticipate the mother's unique emotional needs. Besides the typical emotional responses to labor (see chapters 2 and 3), there are some additional emotional hurdles that the woman who has had a disappointing past experience may have to overcome during labor. They are described here, along with suggestions about how you can help:

- *Early labor.* As she gets into labor, the mother may suddenly lose heart. This is her "moment of truth," and she may be flooded with self-doubt. She will need your encouragement and understanding. Review "Getting into Labor," page 41, and "The Slow-to-Start Labor," page 137, for ideas about helping the mother get into labor both mentally and physically.

- *Flashbacks to the previous labor.* At times, the mother may not be able to escape the feeling that her labor is "just like last time," especially if events in the present labor trigger unpleasant associations with the previous labor. This is normal; you can help by acknowledging the similarity of the two labors, by discussing the mother's feelings, and, most important, by reminding her that this is not "last time" but a completely new labor that she must deal with as such.

- *Reaching the point in this labor at which she had the cesarean or other difficulty in the last labor.* Some women feel a great deal of apprehension before they reach this critical point, and are relieved only after it has passed. Try to help the mother with distraction and stress-reduction measures (see "Comfort Measures for Labor," page 95), and then rejoice with her when she has passed beyond her critical point.

A great potential for healing and growth exists when a woman confronts her difficult memories and deals constructively with them. With preparation beforehand and sensitive, capable support during labor—from you, a doula, and a caring, understanding staff—the mother's experience of birth is almost certain to be far more satisfying and fulfilling than her previous experience was.

Incompatibility with the Nurse or Caregiver

One disadvantage of the North American system of maternity care is that the mother is usually cared for by people she has never met. She hardly ever knows her nurses; she scarcely knows her doctor, whom she may have met briefly six or eight times during her pregnancy. And if her own doctor is not on call when she goes into labor, she will be assisted by a substitute doctor who may be a complete stranger. The kind of care given by some midwives is an exception: Spending time getting to know the mother is one of the features of good midwifery.

Unfortunately, some midwives' practices today have some of the same shortcomings as doctors' practices.

Most of the time no serious problems arise, and the mother, her caregiver, and the nurses get along quite well. What do you do, though, if one or both of you is uncomfortable with the nurse or caregiver? Differences in attitudes toward childbirth, in personality, or in perceptions of each other's roles sometimes become obvious during labor. Discomfort or friction may arise. This *never* works in the mother's best interests. She needs to be surrounded by kind people who she believes will encourage and support her.

If, before labor, you or the mother anticipates problems, be sure to prepare and discuss a Birth Plan. And consider hiring a doula to work with the two of you ahead of time and during labor—to help smooth relations with the staff and to help you and the mother advocate for yourselves.

Usually, problems with the staff are not serious and can easily be resolved. The following are some suggestions for avoiding, minimizing, or solving conflicts:

- Do not be the cause of any friction yourself. By your attitude and your behavior show that you are friendly, respectful, and polite, that you expect to work well with the staff, and that you appreciate their experience and the contributions they can make to the mother's comfort and well-being. If you appear suspicious, frightened, or hostile, the staff might react defensively.
- Make an effort to communicate any special concerns you or the mother have—for example, a desire for natural childbirth, a fear of needles or blood, and so forth.
- Have a copy of the mother's Birth Plan at hand for the nurse to read. If there is time, discuss the Birth Plan with the nurse or caregiver, and ask for help in following the plan as closely as possible. If a staff member has any concerns about the Birth Plan, it is better to discuss these concerns than to ignore them. Differences can usually be resolved easily.
- Call the nurse or caregiver by name.

If there are differences between you or the mother and the nurse, try one or more of the following tactics:

- Deal with the nurse politely. Say, for example, "I cannot talk with you during contractions because I need to help [the mother] breathe and relax"; or "I think there is a misunderstanding. Our doctor said it would be fine for [the mother] to walk around and use the shower. Would you please check with her doctor?"
- Talk to the head nurse. Explain any differences you and the nurse have in a nonaccusatory way and ask the head nurse to assign another nurse or to help mediate the problem.
- Talk directly to the mother's caregiver. If there is an apparent misunderstanding over the nurse's management of labor, ask the caregiver to take care of it. You may have to call the caregiver, if he or she is not in the hospital.

If the problem is with the doctor or midwife (especially if this is someone the mother has never met before), you can try to discuss it directly. If this doesn't solve the problem, ask the nurse to intervene on the mother's behalf and to advocate for her. Or, if the problem involves a clinical decision, ask for a thorough explanation or a second opinion.

Balance the stress that a confrontation will cause against the amount of emotional or physical discomfort resulting from the current arrangement. Sometimes the best interests of the mother are served by avoiding conflict rather than by resolving it—in other words, you may have to accept a less-than-ideal arrangement and work with it.

If you are stuck with a nurse or caregiver with whom you are incompatible and who will not yield, you should accept the situation for the moment and focus your energies on helping the mother cope. You may feel powerless and frustrated under these circumstances, but you cannot stop labor while the problem gets settled. And trying to correct a serious communication problem in the midst of labor might make the labor harder and more stressful for the mother. After the baby is born, you can pursue the matter in an effort to satisfy your frustration and to enlighten those responsible for patient care. While this effort will probably not benefit the mother, baby, or yourself, your efforts may help prevent similar difficulties for another laboring woman in the future.

INCOMPATIBILITY WITH THE NURSE OR CAREGIVER

Part Three

THE MEDICAL SIDE
OF CHILDBIRTH

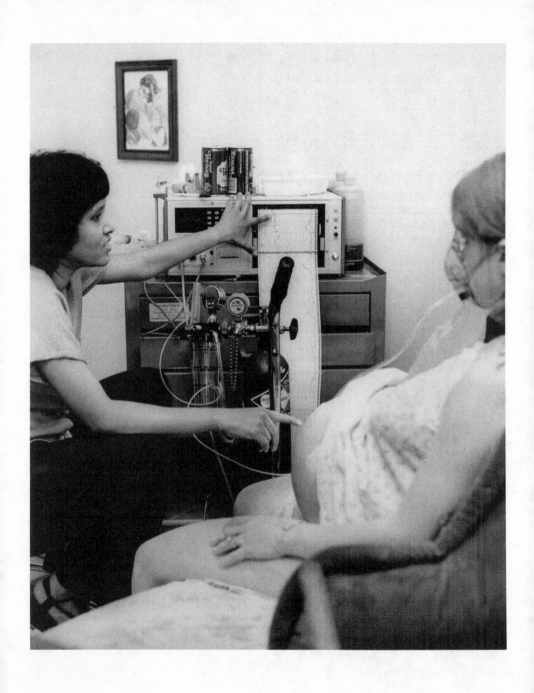

THE CAREGIVER'S PRIMARY ROLE IN CHILDBIRTH is to safeguard the health of mother and child. Throughout pregnancy, the caregiver relies on a wide assortment of tests, technologies, and procedures to detect and treat problems before they become serious. Similar tests and technologies are available during childbirth.

Caregivers differ among themselves regarding what should constitute routine basic care during childbirth. Some caregivers use many medical procedures and interventions in every labor; others use them only when problems are suspected or detected. Pregnant women differ among themselves over the same issue. Some feel more secure with a highly medical approach, while others are wary of this approach, preferring to place more trust in their bodies and their inner resources.

Research has shown that, for a healthy woman, labor proceeds normally and without hazard most of the time, and that careful observation is all that is necessary to detect problems in time to take medical action. Actually, one way to *avoid* problems is to be cautious about using optional procedures and medications; these can sometimes *cause* problems. For example, any procedure that restricts the mother's freedom to move might slow labor or increase her pain, thus making further interventions more likely and actually increasing her risk of developing other problems. In summary, technology, medications, and interventions are appropriate and necessary only when problems already exist or are very likely to occur.

Tests and interventions always involve tradeoffs. The mother needs to know what she gives up and what she gains before making a decision. When considering interventions, discuss the following questions with each other and with the caregiver.

Key Questions
for Informed Decision Making

When a test is suggested, ask

- What is the reason for the test? What questions will it answer?
- How is the test done?

171

- How accurate or reliable are the results? Is there a margin of error? In other words, might the test miss a problem that exists, or identify a problem that does not exist?
- If the test detects a problem, what happens next (for example, further testing, or immediate treatment)?
- If the test does not detect a problem, what happens next (for example, a repeat test in a day or two, other tests, or no further concern about the problem)?
- What will this test cost the mother, if anything?

When a treatment is suggested, ask

- What is the problem, and how serious is it?
- How urgent is the need to begin treatment?
- What is the treatment, and how is it done?
- How likely is it to solve the problem?
- If the treatment fails, what are the next steps?
- Are there any side effects to the treatment?
- Are there any alternatives (including waiting, doing nothing, or other treatments)?

If an alternative is suggested, again ask how it is done, how likely it is to work, what its side effects are, and what happens if the treatment fails.

In most situations, there is plenty of time to discuss these questions. In an emergency, however, there may not be time. The caregiver should tell you how serious and urgent the situation is.

Chapters 6 through 9 discuss the tests, technologies, interventions (including cesarean birth), and medications commonly used in childbirth, along with the problems they are designed to detect and treat.

6

Tests, Technologies, Interventions, and Procedures

What constitutes basic care during the labor of the low-risk mother, that is, the mother who is in good general health, who is experiencing a normal pregnancy, and whose baby is in a favorable position within the uterus? By making certain simple but essential observations regularly during the labor, the skilled caregiver can accurately assess whether the mother and baby are fine or if closer observation or treatment are needed.

Essential Observations

Basic care includes the following essential observations of the mother, the amniotic fluid (the water in the bag of waters), the fetus, and the newborn.

The caregiver makes these observations of the mother:

- Her behavior, activity, and emotional state during and be-tween contractions and after the birth.

- Her basic body functions: eating, drinking, urination, bowel movements.
- Her contractions: their frequency, intensity, and duration, and the tone of the uterus between contractions.
- Her vaginal secretions.
- The progress of labor (determined by the pattern of contractions and by occasional vaginal exams).
- Her vital signs: temperature, pulse, and respiration.
- Her blood pressure.
- The tone of her uterus after childbirth.
- The amount of bleeding after childbirth.

When the bag of water breaks, the caregiver makes these observations of the amniotic fluid:

- The color. Clear means the baby has probably not been stressed; brown or green indicates the presence of fetal bowel movement (meconium), which means the baby is stressed.
- The amount (a leak or a gush). Losing a large amount of fluid increases the likelihood of pressure on the umbilical cord during contractions, which could cause stress to the baby.
- The odor. A foul smell indicates infection.

The caregiver makes these observations of the fetus:

- The heartbeat, monitored by frequent listening to the fetal heart with an ultrasound device or a stethoscope.
- The position (which direction the baby is facing) and the presentation (head down, breech, and so forth).
- The size (approximate weight).

Immediately after birth, the caregiver makes these observations of the newborn:

- The Apgar score (page 175) at 1, 5, and perhaps 10 minutes after birth.
- The baby's temperature, respiration, and pulse.
- The baby's general behavior and state of alertness.
- The baby's physical appearance.

These simple observations, if made frequently by a caregiver who is with the mother continuously or nearly so, give a very good idea of both the mother's condition and the baby's. As

THE APGAR SCORE

Sign	0 points	1 point	2 points
Heart rate	Absent	Below 100 per minute	Over 100 per minute
Breathing	Absent	Slow, irregular	Good, crying
Muscle tone	Limp	Arms and legs close to body	Active, moving
Reflex irritability	No response to suctioning	Grimace	Struggle, cough, or sneeze
Color	Blue-gray	Body pink or ruddy, fingers and toes blue	All pink or ruddy

long as normal conditions are indicated, these observations are all that are truly needed. One-to-one care of the mother by the caregiver or nurse, and the continuous presence of the birth partner and other supporters, allows for kindness, expert emotional support, reassurance, and help with pain-relieving measures at all times. Being with the mother continuously also allows the caregiver or nurse to make other important but less tangible observations about the labor, the mother, or the baby.

In many busy hospitals, continuous one-to-one care from a nurse is impossible. Instead, each nurse cares for two or three laboring women at a time. Each mother has periodic contact with a variety of nurses and doctors, and there is greater reliance on technological substitutes (electronic fetal monitors, intravenous fluid pumps, pain medications, and anesthesia) that allow the nurses to care for more women.

The two approaches result in about the same proportion of healthy mothers and babies. The difference lies more in how these outcomes are achieved. The two approaches can be combined, of course: Continuous nursing and emotional support can be offered along with technology and interventions. This combination is the safest and most effective way to care for mothers who are at moderate or high risk for having problems during labor.

Conditions Influencing
the Amount of Intervention

Beyond the essential observations, many tests, procedures, and medications constitute the medical side of childbirth. They involve the use of highly specialized equipment, a variety of drugs, and surgery. How and when they are used depends on a number of considerations:

- *The medical condition of the mother.* As I have already noted, there is less need for intervention when the mother has had a healthy pregnancy and labor is progressing well.
- *The apparent well-being of the fetus.* If the fetus is fully developed and mature, of normal size, and apparently unstressed, most routine interventions are not needed.
- *The training and philosophy of the caregiver.* Some caregivers routinely use more interventions than others, preferring to treat problems before they arise. Although this practice often results in unnecessary treatment, these caregivers feel that the overtreatment is harmless, and that without it they would miss problems. Better safe than sorry, they believe. Other caregivers are comfortable watching the mother and baby progress, and using treatment only if a problem arises.
- *The usual practices or policies of the institution and nursing staff.* These practices or policies are determined by current standards of care, nurses' training, the size and competence of the staff, customs, medicolegal concerns, financial constraints, and other factors.
- *The preferences of the mother.* Within each institution and within each caregiver's practice, there is room for choice. Be sure the caregiver knows the mother's preferences (see "Review the Mother's Birth Plan," page 25); try to ensure that her preferences are considered in all of the decisions that are made.

Common Obstetric Interventions

Following are descriptions of many common obstetric procedures and their purposes, disadvantages, and possible alternatives. These are usually optional when labor is normal, but they may become necessary if problems arise. Chapter 7, "Problems That May Arise in Late Pregnancy, Labor, or Afterwards," discusses the circumstances under which these procedures are necessary for medical reasons.

As her birth partner, you will be the liaison between the mother and the hospital staff. It is important for you to be familiar with these interventions so that you can inform the staff about the mother's preferences, help the mother make decisions about optional procedures, and help her handle any additional discomfort—emotional or physical—that may arise from the interventions. It is also important for you to make sure the mother understands any changes in her labor that make particular interventions necessary for safety.

Intravenous (IV) Fluids

An intravenous drip is a plastic bag of special liquids containing water, with electrolytes, dextrose, or medications. The bag hangs from a pole attached to the bed or a pole on wheels; the latter allows the mother to walk. A tube extending from the bag is inserted into a vein in the mother's hand or arm. The liquid drips into the vein.

Purposes of Giving IV Fluids. Intravenous fluids may be given (1) to provide the mother liquids, calories, or both, instead of having her drink them; (2) to administer medications; or (3) with an epidural, to increase her blood volume to protect against a drop in blood pressure; or (4) to keep a vein open, just in case the mother requires medications later on.

Many caregivers give intravenous fluids to all their patients in labor, because they do not want these women to eat or drink anything. They feel an empty stomach is best. Their reason dates from the time when most women gave birth while unconscious under general anesthesia. It was dangerous for a woman to have a full stomach while under general anesthesia because she might vomit and breathe in the vomited material. The policy of giving all mothers IVs is continued by many caregivers today, even though general anesthesia is now rarely used for childbirth and,

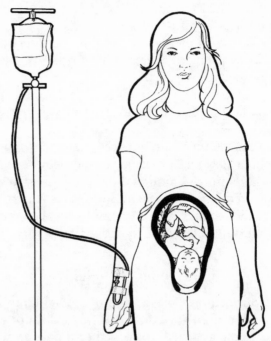

A woman receiving intravenous (IV) fluids.

when it is, better techniques help protect the patient from this complication.

Some caregivers have a less positive attitude toward intravenous fluids. They believe intravenous fluids are problematic much of the time, and they encourage mothers to meet their need for fluids by drinking enough to satisfy their thirst. Intravenous fluids are reserved for times when they are "medically indicated"—that is, when they are necessary or desirable because of the medical condition of the mother or baby.

When are IV fluids medically indicated?

- When labor is very long.
- When the mother has continuous nausea and vomiting.
- When she will receive regional or general anesthesia (page 228).
- When she needs certain IV medications—to stop preterm labor, to induce or augment labor, to control blood pressure, to reduce pain, or for another reason.

- When she has a condition that might require immediate medical action.

Disadvantages of Giving IV Fluids. These are

- IV fluids in large amounts may cause temporary low blood sugar (if the fluids contain dextrose, a type of sugar), or electrolyte imbalance (if the fluids contain electrolytes) in the baby soon after birth.
- Large amounts of IV fluids cause fluid retention in the mother, especially in her legs and breasts, which takes days to disappear. Rarely, excess fluid accumulates in the mother's lungs (this is called pulmonary edema).
- An IV line is inconvenient and somewhat stressful for the mother, who must make sure it is out of the way as she rolls over or gets out of bed.
- IV lines sometimes "infiltrate," that is, they poke through the vein. The fluids then go directly into the mother's tissue, causing pain and swelling. If the fluids contain medications, they do no good, since they do not get into her bloodstream.
- IV fluids are unnecessary if the mother drinks enough liquid and does not need intravenous medication. She requires about ¼ cup liquid per hour, or somewhat more if she is sweating a lot or doing mostly light breathing. The best policy is usually to encourage her to drink when she feels thirsty.

Alternatives to Consider. You and the mother can discuss the following alternatives with the mother's caregiver:

- If labor is proceeding rapidly, do not give the mother any IV fluids; the mother may get along without any fluids, by vein or by mouth.
- Give the mother fluids to drink, such as water, fruit juice, or sports beverages (with their added electrolytes) or frozen juice bars to eat. It is a good idea for her to drink something after each contraction or two.
- Keep a vein open (in case of emergency, if the mother is worried about this) without giving IV fluids. To do this, the caregiver places a needle in a vein in the mother's arm above her wrist, but the needle is plugged and not connected to an intravenous line. This procedure (called a *heparin lock*)

allows the mother more freedom to move around than does an intravenous line. It also allows the caregiver to give intravenous medications very quickly if the need arises.

Electronic Fetal Monitoring (EFM)

There are two methods of electronic fetal monitoring (EFM), external and internal.

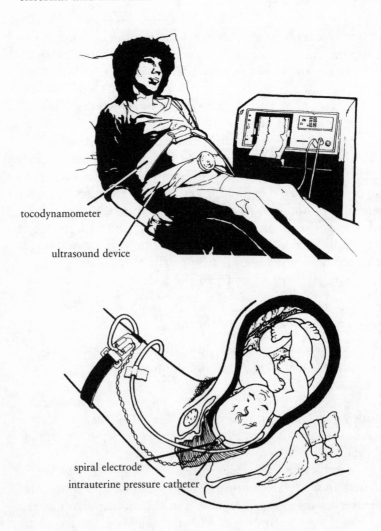

Electronic fetal monitoring (EFM): external (above) and internal (below).

With external monitoring, the nurse or caregiver places two stretchy belts around the mother's abdomen. One holds an ultrasound device in the best place to detect the fetal heartbeat. It is placed low on the woman's abdomen. The other, placed higher, holds a device (a *tocodynamometer*) that detects contractions.

With internal fetal monitoring, a thin, spiral wire electrode is placed in the skin of the baby's scalp to detect the fetal heart rate. And a fluid-filled plastic tube (an intrauterine pressure catheter) is placed within the mother's uterus to detect and measure the intensity of the contractions. When the uterus contracts, fluid is squeezed out of the tube, and a gauge measures the strength of the contraction. Both external and internal monitoring devices are connected by wires to a calibrating and recording machine that flashes numbers every second on a digital display, indicating both fetal heart rate and tone in the uterus. These readings are continuously printed out on paper, in graph form, and are transmitted to a monitor at the nurses' station. Some partners find the monitor helpful as a guide for when a contraction is beginning.

The external methods are easier to apply, less invasive, and much more widely used than the internal methods, which are reserved for times when external monitoring is not tracking the fetal heartbeat or the contractions accurately enough.

Purposes of EFM. Before labor, EFM is used to assess the fetus's well-being through the nonstress test, which assesses the response of the fetal heart rate when the fetus moves. The mother indicates when she feels her baby move by pressing a button. If the heart rate speeds up, this is a good sign; if it stays the same or slows down, the fetus may be stressed, and further tests or corrective action may be necessary.

During labor, EFM is used to help the caregiver or nurse assess the fetus's response to labor and the adequacy of uterine contractions.

When is EFM medically indicated?

- When there are doubts before labor about the fetus's well-being.
- When labor is prolonged and the caregiver is considering speeding progress by administering oxytocin. The length and

frequency of the contractions can be assessed with the external tocodynamometer. If the caregiver needs to know the intensity of the contractions, the intrauterine pressure catheter is used.

- When a nurse or a midwife cannot remain with the mother continuously.
- When the mother receives oxytocin or other medications that might affect the fetus.
- When there are doubts during labor about the fetus's well-being (because of prematurity, small size, or possible lack of oxygen).
- When the mother is considered to be at high risk for complications.

Disadvantages of EFM. These are

- The mother's movements are restricted, although she can change position in bed and sometimes even stand by the bed or sit in a chair. Internal monitoring is less restrictive than external.
- Sometimes more attention is paid to the machine than to the mother. As her birth partner, do not allow yourself to fall into this trap.
- Interpretation of the monitor printouts (tracings) is extremely complex, and experts disagree about what different heart-rate patterns really mean and when intervention is necessary.
- Internal monitoring requires both breaking the bag of waters and breaking the skin of the fetal scalp. These procedures slightly increase the risk of infection to mother and baby, especially if the mother has an infection or sore in her vagina. Also, breaking the bag of waters may cause additional stress to the fetus because it removes the cushion of fluid that protects the head and cord.
- EFM measures only the fetal pulse, not actual fetal distress—that is, a shortage of oxygen. When a cesarean is done solely because of EFM tracings, the baby may show no signs of having suffered fetal distress. For this reason, other tests have been developed to confirm the findings of EFM (see "Fetal Stimulation Test," page 184, and "Fetal Oxygen Saturation Monitoring," page 184).

Alternatives to Consider. You and the mother can discuss the following alternatives to EFM with the mother's caregiver:

- Have a nurse or caregiver listen frequently to fetal heart tones with an ultrasound stethoscope or a fetal stethoscope, for 1 to 2 minutes at a time during and after a contraction. Many studies have compared this method of monitoring with continuous EFM, and all have found that having a nurse listen to heart tones intermittently results in equally healthy babies and fewer cesareans. This method does, however, require continuous attendance by a skilled nurse or midwife.

- Use intermittent external EFM for 10 to 15 minutes each hour. This enables the mother to move around the rest of the time.

- Use a portable radio-transmission (telemetry) EFM unit. The mother wears the unit on a belt, which allows her to move about freely (within about 200 feet of the nurses' station) while information is radioed back to a central monitor. Find out if the hospital has telemetry units available.

- Use a waterproof ultrasound stethoscope for listening to the baby when the mother is in the bath.

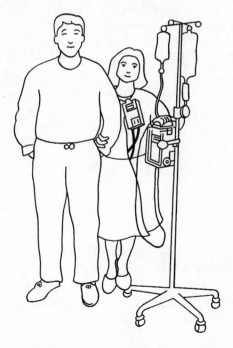

Fetal Stimulation Test

The caregiver performs this simple test by pressing or scratching the fetal scalp during a vaginal exam (the fetal scalp stimulation test) or, less commonly, by making a loud noise outside the uterus (the fetal acoustic stimulation test). If the fetus is in good condition, the heart rate will speed up with such stimulation. If the fetus is distressed (that is, short of oxygen), the heart rate will not speed up. The results of this test have been found to correlate well with the more complex, expensive, and time-consuming fetal oxygen saturation monitoring, described later.

Purposes of the Fetal Stimulation Test. This test is performed to confirm whether the fetus is truly in distress when EFM or monitoring by stethoscope suggests that he may be. The test is medically indicated any time fetal distress is suspected, and certainly before a cesarean is performed for fetal distress.

Disadvantages of the Fetal Stimulation Test. There are none.

Alternatives to Consider. The alternatives to performing the fetal stimulation test include the following: (1) relying on EFM alone; (2) relying on frequent listening to the fetal heart rate alone; or (3) relying on EFM plus fetal oxygen saturation monitoring (see the discussion that follows). None of these provides an advantage over the fetal stimulation test; the first two result in more false diagnoses and unnecessary treatment of fetal distress, and the last is far more expensive and cumbersome.

You and the mother can ask for the fetal stimulation test whenever fetal distress is suspected. Discuss it with her caregiver in advance, and state your preference for it in her Birth Plan (page 25).

Fetal Oxygen Saturation Monitoring (FOSM)

This procedure can be added to electronic fetal monitoring to check more closely when EFM indicates that the fetal heart-rate pattern is "nonreassuring," that is, it indicates that the baby may not be getting enough oxygen. FOSM involves the insertion of an oxygenation sensor (a flexible plate the size of a Band-aid) through the cervix. Connected by a wire to the monitor console, the sensor is placed alongside the baby's cheek, where it detects the amount of oxygen in the baby's blood. The "oxygen saturation" is measured as a percentage of the maximum amount of oxygen possible. Above 30 percent indicates the fetus is doing well, even if the heart rate is concerning. The monitor console continuously records the oxygen saturation, and the printout is checked periodically by the nurse to detect any change.

FOSM and the fetal stimulation tests have largely replaced an older test called fetal scalp blood sampling, which, though helpful in identifying true fetal distress, was slow, cumbersome, and more invasive than the two newer tests.

An advantage over the fetal stimulation test is that FOSM provides a continuous record of fetal oxygen saturation, instead of periodic assessments.

As a more direct measure of fetal well-being than electronic fetal monitoring, FOSM may reduce the number of cesareans for fetal distress. But since the procedure has only recently been introduced, discovering its true value and cost-effectiveness may take years.

Disadvantages of FOSM. These are

- FOSM is very expensive compared to the fetal stimulation test, which costs nothing. Each single-use sensor costs one to two hundred dollars, and if it is placed incorrectly or it becomes covered with the baby's vernix (a creamy coating on the skin), it has to be discarded and replaced.
- The sensor must be placed flat against the baby's cheek, which is challenging as it must be done by feel.
- Before FOSM can be used, the membranes must be ruptured and the cervix partially dilated. If the membranes have not ruptured spontaneously, the caregiver ruptures them artificially (see page 187).

Group B Strep (GBS) Screening

This is a test for the presence of particular bacteria, called Group B Streptococci, in the mother's urine, rectum, or vagina. Offered in late pregnancy at a prenatal appointment, the test involves culturing a sample of secretions from her vagina or rectum. Results are usually available in two to three days, although a rapid test, which gives results within minutes, is used by some hospitals when women arrive with ruptured membranes.

One in three to four pregnant women is a "carrier" of GBS, which means that the bacteria are present in her body fluids, but she shows no signs of infection. Approximately 1 to 2 percent of babies born to these women acquire a GBS infection, which can be extremely serious for the newborn. As preventive treatment, antibiotics are given to the mother after her membranes rupture. The antibiotics reach the baby via the placenta, lowering the risk of newborn infection substantially. The antibiotics also lower the mother's risk of developing a GBS infection.

If a GBS carrier delivers before she has received sufficient antibiotics, her baby will probably be tested (with a complete blood culture, possibly a urine culture, and possibly a spinal tap and culture of spinal fluid) and treated with intravenous antibiotics for two to three days, until the tests are complete. If the tests show that the baby is uninfected, all treatment stops. But if Group B Strep bacteria are present in the cultures, the antibiotic treatment continues for many days, during which the baby must remain in the hospital.

The main disadvantage of GBS screening is that, if a woman is found to be a carrier, she faces an increased likelihood of induction of labor if her membranes rupture and her contractions do not begin within a reasonable length of time. Some women do not go into labor for days after their membranes rupture. Many caregivers, and many of their patients, question the wisdom of giving numerous doses of antibiotics during the waiting period. A common practice is to give a maximum of four doses, and to suggest induction if the mother does not go into labor within 24 hours. Some caregivers are more patient than others under these circumstances, as are some women. Either choice—large amounts of antibiotics over time, or induction—has disadvantages (see page 193).

Artificial Rupture of the Membranes (AROM)

To rupture the membranes, the caregiver inserts a long thin instrument (amnihook) into the vagina and painlessly breaks the bag of waters. The "waters" (amniotic fluid) come out in a gush or a stream. Sometimes, following AROM, the woman's contractions suddenly increase in intensity. Contrary to previously widespread belief, bathing after the membranes are ruptured does not increase the chance of infection in mother or baby.

Purposes of AROM. AROM is done

- To speed labor. If timed correctly, it often succeeds in shortening labor by an average of 40 minutes.
- To induce labor with or without other methods, such as prostaglandin gel or oxytocin induction (see page 190). AROM is not likely to succeed, however, unless the cervix is very soft and thin.
- To check the amniotic fluid for a fetal bowel movement (that is, for the presence of meconium, which signals fetal stress), for infection, for bleeding, or for other signs of problems.
- To apply the electrode and catheter for internal EFM, or the sensor for fetal oxygen saturation monitoring.

When is AROM medically indicated? This question is controversial. The frequency with which caregivers use AROM, especially in early labor, varies widely. Some believe it is in-

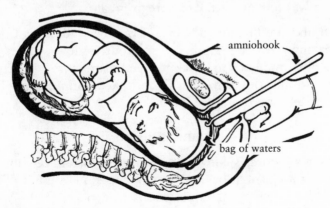

amniohook

bag of waters

Artificial rupture of the membranes.

nocuous and use it for most of their patients in labor. Others believe its advantages rarely outweigh its disadvantages; they reserve it for situations where they feel they must intervene. Otherwise, they prefer to leave the membranes intact.

Disadvantages of AROM. These are

- Frequently, it does not speed labor.
- The chances of the mother or the baby getting an infection are increased if the bag of waters remains broken for a long time before birth, especially if vaginal exams are performed.
- Removing the protective cushion of fluid from around the fetal head may increase pressure on the head during contractions and thus cause more head molding, the gradual and temporary reshaping of the baby's head that results from pressures within the birth canal. A certain amount of molding is normal and desirable, because it enables the head to pass through a small, tight space. Excessive molding, however, may cause damage to the fetal skull.
- AROM also increases the risk that the umbilical cord will be compressed during contractions, which could cause a lack of oxygen for the fetus.
- If the baby's head (or buttocks, if the baby is breech) is high when AROM is done, the danger of prolapsed cord (page 213) increases.

Alternatives to Consider. The caregiver can

- Refrain from breaking the bag of waters at all or wait before breaking it to see if labor will speed up on its own.
- Use other methods to check for fetal distress (see "Electronic Fetal Monitoring," page 180, and "Fetal Stimulation Test," page 184) and to induce labor.

Amnioinfusion

In this procedure, saline (salty water) is introduced into the uterus via a plastic tube, the same one used in internal EFM to assess the intensity of contractions (see page 180). Amnioinfusion is done after the bag of waters has broken, if the baby's umbilical cord is being compressed during contractions. The added fluid helps to cushion the cord and may protect against fetal distress. The procedure also is helpful if the baby has passed meconium in the uterus. The fluid dilutes the meconium to protect against problems that would occur if the baby were to inhale thick meconium during birth. Although the injected fluid gradually runs out of the uterus, the procedure can be repeated as necessary to maintain a sufficient volume. This simple technique, which is extremely low in cost, sometimes makes it possible to safely avoid a cesarean for fetal distress.

Disadvantages of Amnioinfusion. These are the following:

- It is invasive.
- It requires that the membranes be ruptured.
- The mother cannot be upright, or the fluid would run out quickly. She must lie in bed.

Alternatives to Consider. The caregiver can

- Refrain from breaking the bag of waters. Artificial rupture of the membranes is often the cause of cord compression.

Induction or Augmentation of Labor

Sometimes labor is induced (artificially started); at other times a labor that has slowed down is speeded up (augmented). There are several ways labor can be induced or augmented:

1. Self-help methods (see pages 147–152).
2. Stripping the membranes to begin labor induction. The caregiver inserts a finger into the cervix and circles around the inside to separate the membranes from the lower segment of the uterus. This is usually painful for the mother—it feels like a very vigorous vaginal exam—and it sometimes results in inadvertent rupture of the membranes. Stripping the membranes usually does not actually start labor, but it may hasten changes in the cervix to prepare it for dilation (see "Labor Progresses in Six Ways," page 50). The procedure cannot be done if the cervical opening is hard to reach because it is very posterior (pointing toward the mother's back) instead of anterior (in the center of her vagina), and if it is tightly closed.

3. Artificial rupture of the membranes (AROM). This sometimes speeds or augments labor, if it is timed correctly (see the preceding discussion).

4. Prostaglandins promote the softening, thinning, and, sometimes, dilation of the cervix. These hormone-like substances are used when labor must be induced before the cervix has naturally softened or thinned. Prostaglandins come in a variety of forms:

- A gel (Prepidil) that is applied within or outside the cervix through a syringe. More may be applied after six hours or so.
- A tampon-like device (Cervidil) that gradually releases prostaglandin over about 12 hours. The device is placed in the vagina behind the cervix.
- A tiny tablet (Cytotec) that is usually placed in the vagina behind the cervix, but is sometimes given to the mother by mouth. A second tablet may be administered after three hours. Cytotec is much more likely to cause contractions and dilation than is Prepidil or Cervidil.

Dosages and treatment schedules vary depending on the caregiver's preferences, the woman's preferences, and the state of her cervix.

5. Intravenous administration of the hormone oxytocin (also called Pitocin). This can start or speed up labor. The oxytocin is mixed with intravenous fluids; a continuous intravenous drip causes uterine contractions. By regulating the dose, the caregiver can usually control the intensity and frequency of the contractions quite well. Electronic fetal monitoring (EFM) is required, along with a nurse's close observation, to detect and correct excessively strong or long contractions. Attempts to start labor with oxytocin often fail when the cervix is firm and thick. If prostaglandin is used before oxytocin, this problem is often avoided. If the induction fails, cesarean delivery is the only remaining option.

Purposes of Induction or Augmentation. Induction or augmentation of labor is medically indicated

- When pregnancy is prolonged. Caregivers disagree about when pregnancy has gone on too long. Some offer induction at 40 or 41 weeks, but most agree that risks to the baby begin to

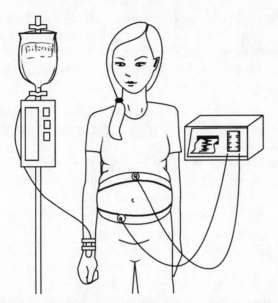

The mother is having her labor induced with Pitocin. Her contractions and the fetal heart rate are being monitored electronically.

increase by 42 weeks and will induce labor at that time. Some caregivers wait for warning signs of problems with the mother or the baby before suggesting induction. For these caregivers, the length of pregnancy, by itself, is not a major consideration.

- When medical problems are such that continuing the pregnancy might harm the mother or the baby (for example, when the mother has high blood pressure, diabetes, or some other condition).
- When the baby is not thriving in the uterus.
- Sometimes when the bag of waters has been broken for a long time and labor has not started spontaneously, or the mother has tested positive for Group B Strep (see page 185).
- When the mother is having a prolonged prelabor and her cervix is firm, in which case the use of prostaglandin gel may be appropriate (see "Prelabor," page 60, and "The Slow-to-Start Labor," page 137).
- When contractions in the active phase slow down and decrease in intensity, causing a delay in progress, augmentation may be appropriate.

Sometimes labor is induced out of fear that the baby is becoming too big. The reasoning is that inducing labor before the baby grows too much makes the birth easier and prevents complications and a possible cesarean. Although this seems to make sense, studies have shown

- It is not possible to accurately assess an unborn baby's size. Estimates are often wrong by 10 percent even when ultrasound is used.
- Most babies who do not fit through the pelvis and birth canal are of average size or smaller. Their position within the uterus and the shape of the mother's pelvis, which cannot be improved by induction, are the cause.
- When babies are thought to be large, cesareans are actually more likely if labor is induced than if labor begins spontaneously, and induction in these cases produces no improvements in the babies' health and well-being.
- Although the odds of a difficult labor increase when the baby's weight exceeds 8½ pounds, inducing labor does not prevent a difficult labor or a cesarean birth.

Nonmedical Reasons for Induction. Most inductions done today are "elective"; that is, they are done not for medical safety but for such reasons as

- Convenience for the mother, her caregiver, or both. An elective induction may be scheduled to occur when the caregiver is on call or when the mother has household help.
- Routine procedure, whenever a mother reaches her fortieth week. Many caregivers see no reason not to induce labor at this point.
- The mother's discomfort. Swelling, backache, or fatigue makes some women want to end their pregnancies as soon as safety allows.
- Avoiding the stress of going to the hospital in labor, especially if the mother lives far from the hospital or has had a previous rapid labor.
- Avoiding entering labor with a herpes sore, in hopes of avoiding a cesarean, if the mother has frequent herpes outbreaks. A cesarean is done if a woman has a herpes sore in or

near her vagina when she goes in to labor.

It can be very appealing for the mother to be able to plan when the baby will be born. And, as her birth partner, you might also appreciate knowing the date and being able to plan your schedule around it. Most inductions proceed well, especially if they are done when the cervix has already ripened (softened and thinned) considerably. The staff usually tries to avoid the sudden onset of painful contractions by starting with low doses of medication and increasing them gradually. Cytotec (misoprostol), the newest induction agent, is the most difficult to control; with it, the contractions sometimes suddenly becoming overwhelming (in 2000, the manufacturer of this ulcer medication expressed concern over the use of the drug for inducing labor—a purpose for which it was never intended).

Because induction is not an innocuous procedure, the benefits and risks of an elective induction should be carefully considered before a decision is made. There are many potential disadvantages:

1. Inductions often proceed very slowly, especially if the mother's cervix has not undergone some of the pre-dilation changes (see "Labor Progresses in Six Ways," page 50). Days may pass before the baby is born, so the induction procedures are carried out during the day and stopped at night to allow the woman to eat and get some rest. The reason for allowing plenty of time for the process is to try to avoid a cesarean; however, a slow induction can be exhausting and demoralizing for both the mother and the birth partner. (If the bag of waters has broken, the caregiver usually intervenes with a cesarean earlier.)

2. The timing of an elective induction may not be best for the baby, who might benefit from another few days in the uterus. Most babies continue to mature and develop greater strength and other capabilities until labor begins spontaneously. If the mother's due date is uncertain, the baby might actually be born prematurely if labor is induced.

3. Prostaglandins sometimes cause nausea in the mother and rapid changes in her blood pressure.

4. The chances of a cesarean increase markedly in first-time mothers who have elective inductions.

5. Sometimes, even though the induction date is planned, the hospital is too busy or no bed is available when the day comes. The mother may be asked to call the hospital every few hours to see if a bed is available. This can be frustrating, especially if she has not been warned in advance that this could happen.

6. Induced labors may cause contractions that are too long or too strong for the baby (or the mother) to tolerate. To detect such a problem, the mother is subjected to continuous electronic fetal monitoring (see page 180). If her contractions are too strong and the baby is not tolerating them well, the nurse may take measures to stop the contractions. If the mother is receiving intravenous oxytocin, the nurse can turn it off; the oxytocin leaves the mother's bloodstream very quickly, so the contractions usually quickly subside. If the mother has had prostaglandin placed in her vagina, the nurse either removes the insert (Cervidil) or gives a douche to wash out the gel (Prepidil) or the tablet (Cytotec). If the mother has swallowed a Cytotec tablet, there is no way to remove it, so another drug, such as Terbutaline, may be given to slow the contractions.

7. Use of pain medications early in the dilation process is more likely with induction, for several reasons:

- The mother may be restricted by the intravenous drip and the electronic fetal monitor from using comfort measures such as position changes, movements, and massage.
- Fatigue and discouragement over a slow onset of labor may lower the mother's motivation to deal with her contractions. She also may feel hungry, since she will probably not be allowed to eat while the oxytocin is being given.
- Following induction, from the time labor begins until the cervix has dilated a few centimeters, the contractions come closer and last longer than they would if labor began spontaneously.
- If the mother is hospitalized before contractions start, the labor seems much longer and slower than it would if labor began at home where she could continue normal activities and keep busy.

A medically indicated induction has some of the same disadvantages, but knowing a clear reason for the induction may make the disadvantages easier to accept.

Alternatives to Consider. Instead of having labor medically induced or augmented you can

- Wait for spontaneous labor. If the mother asks about postponing an elective induction, she will probably find that her caregiver is willing to wait for labor to start on its own—so long as there is careful surveillance of the mother's and fetus's well-being. If, however, the caregiver feels the baby must be born soon, for a medical reason, the mother should take the caregiver's opinions very seriously.
- Try the nonmedical methods for stimulating labor contractions described on pages 147 to 152, "When Labor Must Start."

Episiotomy

An episiotomy is a surgical cut, made with scissors, from the vagina toward the anus. It is sometimes done shortly before delivery. Anesthesia may be given before the procedure, although even if the episiotomy is done without anesthesia, the mother is hardly aware of it. Rather than feeling pain, she is aware of a relief from pressure when the episiotomy is performed. Local anesthesia is given after the birth to relieve pain that occurs when the episiotomy is stitched. The incision usually heals

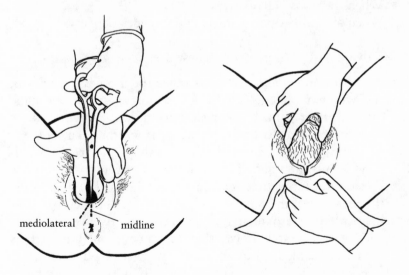

mediolateral   midline

Episiotomy. The midline incision is most common in the United States.

within one or two weeks, although pain at the site occasionally lingers, especially during intercourse, for months. If she still has pain after a few weeks, however, the mother should consult her caregiver.

Once routine, episiotomies are rarely performed by mid-wives, and physicians are doing many fewer than they were in the early and mid-nineties.

Purposes of Episiotomy. These are

- To speed delivery by a few minutes if the fetus appears to be distressed.
- To reduce pressure on the baby's head if the baby is prema-ture or has other problems.
- To try to avoid a tear of the labia (the "lips," or folds of skin, on either side of the vagina) or perineum (the area between the vagina and the anus).
- To allow easier placement of forceps.
- To enlarge a very tight vaginal opening when this is necessary to allow delivery. It is very rare that the vagina will not stretch adequately.

When is an episiotomy medically indicated?

- When the fetus is in distress.
- When a rigid perineum slows and impedes delivery.

Disadvantages of Episiotomy. These are

- An episiotomy will *definitely* damage the mother's perineum; she will have a cut, stitches, a healing period, and some discomfort or pain. If no episiotomy is done, however, there is only about a 30 to 50 percent chance that the mother's perineum will tear. Research indicates that tears are almost al-ways smaller and quicker to heal than the average episiotomy.
- Episiotomies sometimes *extend*—that is, after the cut is made, the pressure of the baby's head can enlarge the incision. This happens in approximately one woman in twenty. Spontan-eous tears are rarely (fewer than one time in one hundred) as large as extended episiotomies. In other words, the chance of a serious tear is greater with an episiotomy than without.

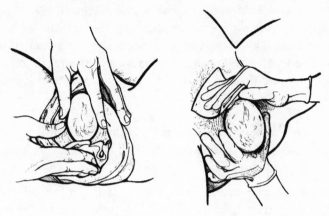

An alternative to episiotomy. Left, *the caregiver uses warm compresses to promote relaxation and circulation, and gently supports the perineum.* Right, *the caregiver provides slight counterpressure as the baby's head emerges.*

Alternatives to Consider. The caregiver can

- Simply forego an episiotomy, even if it appears that the mother may tear. She may incur no injury, one or several small tears, or, rarely, a large tear.
- Protect the perineum from tearing seriously—for example, by placing hot compresses on the perineum, controlling the birth of the head and shoulders, suggesting positions that facilitate the baby's descent, and allowing spontaneous bearing down (see "The Crowning and Birth Phase," page 78, and "Spontaneous Bearing Down," page 110).

The mother can improve her chance of an intact perineum after birth by doing prenatal perineal massage or having you do it for her (see page 21).

Whether or not a woman ends up with a perineal tear or cut, exercising her pelvic floor muscles after birth seems to be most important to the recovery of pelvic floor tone. See pages 20 and 21 for discussions of the Kegel exercise.

Vacuum Extraction

Vacuum extraction is used during the birthing (second) stage of labor. A plastic suction cup (about 3 inches in diameter) is placed on the baby's head; the suction cup is connected to handles and to a pump device that sets the amount of suction at a safe level. The caregiver pulls on the device attached to the baby's head while the uterus contracts and the mother pushes. The suction cup disengages if the caregiver pulls too hard, thus protecting the baby's head.

Purposes of Vacuum Extraction. Vacuum extraction is done to assist or hasten delivery after the baby's head is in the birth canal. It is medically indicated

- If the birthing (second) stage of labor is prolonged because fatigue or anesthesia have made the mother unable to push effectively.
- If the birthing stage is prolonged because the baby's head is slightly angled so that it doesn't fit through the pelvis, and the mother's efforts need assistance.
- If there is last-minute fetal distress.

Compared with forceps (page 199), the vacuum extractor is less likely to require an episiotomy; it may cause less damage to the woman's vagina; it can be used when the baby is higher in the birth canal; and it appears to be about as safe for the baby.

Disadvantages of Vacuum Extraction. These are

- Vacuum extraction frequently causes a fluid-filled lump and a bruise or abrasion on the baby's head where the suction cup

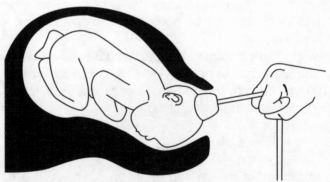

Vacuum extraction. After applying a suction cup to the baby's scalp, the caregiver pulls as the mother pushes and the uterus contracts.

was. It may take days or weeks for the lump to disappear.
- More serious injury to the fetal head is possible, though unlikely when vacuum extraction is used properly.
- If the suction cup pops off during use, both the birth partner and the mother may be alarmed. Remember, it pops off to protect the baby from excessive strain.
- Most midwives and some family physicians are untrained in this technique, and so must call in an obstetrician if vacuum extraction is needed.

Alternatives to Consider. These are

- The mother can bear down (push) in different positions, such as squatting or standing. See "Positions and Movements for Labor and Birth," page 112.
- Forceps can be used for delivery (see below).
- A cesarean section can be performed (see chapter 9).

Forceps Delivery

Forceps are used during the birthing stage. Two steel instruments (like spoons or salad tongs) are placed within the vagina on either

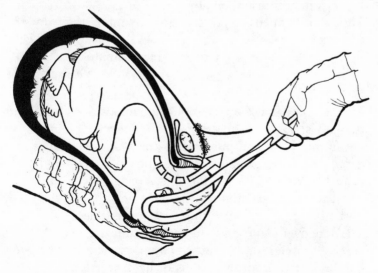

Forceps are placed in the mother's vagina around the baby's head. The doctor pulls while the mother pushes and the uterus contracts.

side of the baby's head. They are then locked into position so they cannot squeeze the baby's head, no matter how hard the doctor grips the handles. This protects the baby's head from undue pressure. The doctor pulls during contractions, while the mother pushes. Sometimes forceps are used to rotate the baby's head.

Purposes of Using Forceps. The doctor uses forceps to deliver the baby more quickly. A forceps delivery is medically indicated

- If the birth is delayed because (1) the mother is not able to push effectively, (2) there is a decrease in uterine contractions, or (3) the baby is large.
- If there is fetal distress when the baby is low in the birth canal.

If the baby is high, either a vacuum extraction or a cesarean delivery (see chapter 9) is a safer choice than forceps. If a forceps delivery appears difficult, the attempt is abandoned, and a cesarean is performed.

Disadvantages of Forceps Delivery. These are

- A forceps delivery usually requires an episiotomy and anesthesia.
- Forceps may bruise the baby's head or face.
- Though it happens rarely, forceps may injure the baby's head or neck.
- Forceps may injure the mother's birth canal.

Alternatives to Consider. These are

- The mother can use directed pushing in positions that enlarge the pelvis, such as squatting or a supported squat, or lying flat on her back and pulling her knees up toward her shoulders. See "Positions and Movements for Labor and Birth," page 112, and "Directed Pushing," page 111.
- The caregiver can monitor the fetus and the mother, and, if both are doing well, give the labor more time.
- The caregiver can use vacuum extraction (see page 198). The choice between forceps and vacuum extraction is best made by the doctor, according to his or her expertise.
- The doctor can perform a cesarean delivery if it appears that a forceps delivery would be difficult (see chapter 9).

7
Problems That May Arise in Late Pregnancy, Labor, or Afterwards

This chapter discusses a number of problems that may arise before, during, or after labor, how they are treated, and how you can help the mother. These problems usually resolve themselves with time or with minor interventions, but occasionally they require rapid action and major interventions, such as cesarean delivery. The problems fall into four major categories: problems with the mother; problems with the labor; problems with the fetus; and problems with the newborn.

As you would imagine, the mother will be upset—worried, shocked, stunned, frightened, anxious, or even suspicious—if problems arise. She may have difficulty accepting that there is a problem, especially if she feels normal. It is awfully hard to cope with much more than labor itself, and she may rely on you to assume some of the responsibility for decision making.

As the birth partner, you can help in the following ways:

- Learn, and help the mother to understand, what is happening, why it is a problem, how serious it is, and the rationale for and the expected results of any corrective action to be taken. Ask her caregiver the key questions on page 171.
- Help the mother adjust to the need for a change in management. She may need help making decisions.
- Remain assertive and cooperative with her caregiver. Ask questions, inform the staff of the mother's wishes, and learn of any alternative ways of handling the problem. Use her Birth Plan (see page 25) as your guide.
- Recognize the need to accept the caregiver's judgment in true emergencies, when time is of the utmost importance.
- Remain with the mother throughout. When things go wrong, she needs your help and support more than ever.
- Afterwards, allow her time to recover emotionally.

Problems with the Mother

Premature Labor

If a woman begins labor before 37 weeks of pregnancy, the labor is considered premature (see "The Signs of Labor," page 45, for an explanation of signs of premature labor). If the baby is born prematurely, he is at greater risk for a number of medical problems, such as breathing difficulties, jaundice, infection, difficulty maintaining body temperature, and feeding problems.

Management of Premature Labor. This depends on the fetus's gestational age, well-being, and stage of development. Measures may include the following:

- A vaginal exam to determine how much the cervix has dilated.
- Assessment of contractions (how long, strong, and frequent they are).
- Attempts to stop labor through the use of bed rest and medications such as terbutaline, magnesium sulfate, ritodrine, nifedipine, or other medications. Treatment is more likely to

be effective if the woman's cervix has not dilated beyond 2 centimeters.

- Amniocentesis and testing of the amniotic fluid to indicate if the fetus's lungs are mature, that is, capable of breathing without difficulty after birth. This helps the caregiver determine how aggressively to try to stop the labor.
- Medications (corticosteroids) given to the mother via injection to hasten the maturation of the baby's lungs, if birth cannot be postponed and the baby's lungs are immature.
- Electronic fetal monitoring (EFM) to detect contractions and to watch the baby's condition.
- A test for infection, which sometimes causes premature labor. The mother must be treated with antibiotics if the test is positive.
- If delivery cannot be postponed, transportation of the mother to a hospital with an intensive-care nursery, especially if the baby will be born very early (at less than 33 weeks gestation).
- Summoning of a pediatrician or neonatologist to care for the baby immediately after the delivery.
- If delivery is postponed, the mother may be sent home on medication and required to lie down all the time until 36 weeks or so.

Mother's Reactions. The mother will be anxious to do all she can to help the baby to a healthy start in life. She may feel guilty about not being able to do her share of housework and meal preparation. She may feel sorry for you and concerned over adding pressure on you. She may worry how a lengthy period of bed rest will affect her strength and fitness (her caregivers may be able to recommend a physical therapist who can visit her and teach her some safe in-bed exercises). She may become bored lying around all the time.

How You Can Help. Try not to add to her feelings of guilt. Consider your added responsibilities as your contribution to your baby's health and well-being. Try to ease your burden by getting household help. Encourage the mother to shop for the baby by catalog or Internet. She might communicate with others on bed rest via the Internet, too. This is also a good time for her to read books and watch videos on baby care and feeding. Her childbirth educator or public library may have such videotapes available.

Rise in the Mother's Blood Pressure

The mother's blood pressure is checked at each prenatal appointment. If it rises significantly (to about 140/90 or higher) she has pregnancy-induced hypertension (PIH), which may be mild to severe. Sometimes mild PIH becomes more severe during labor. If mild, she may also have swelling in her legs, hands, and face, and protein in her urine. If the PIH becomes severe, she may have blurring of or spots in her vision, upper abdominal pain, headaches, increased reflexes (for example, when her knee is tapped, the mother's foot jerks more than usual), and liver and kidney problems (the last are detected by a blood test). The function of her placenta may be impaired, and this may slow the baby's growth. If the PIH is very severe, the mother may experience convulsions, and even death is possible. The complications arising from severe PIH are referred to by the terms *preeclampsia, eclampsia, toxemia,* and *HELLP* syndrome, which stands for hemolysis (breakdown of red blood cells), elevated liver enzymes, and low platelets (which interfered with her body's ability to clot blood).

Management of High Blood Pressure During Pregnancy. Measures may include

- Bed rest, preferably on her left side. The number of hours of bed rest each day depends on the severity of the PIH and the caregiver's belief in the value of bed rest. Opinions vary quite a lot.
- Medications to lower blood pressure (such as hydralazine or nifedipine) or to prevent convulsions (magnesium sulfate).
- Close monitoring of her blood pressure and other signs of worsening PIH (through blood and urine tests, checking of reflexes, tests of fetal growth and well-being, and weight checks).
- Induction of labor or even a cesarean if her condition worsens.

Management of High Blood Pressure During Labor. Measures may include

- Restriction to left-sided bed rest. Some caregivers allow a warm shower or bath from time to time during labor, as these also lower blood pressure.
- Continuous electronic fetal monitoring and intravenous fluids.
- Frequent blood-pressure checks.
- Medications to lower blood pressure and magnesium sulfate to prevent convulsions, if the condition is severe.
- Intravenous oxytocin (Pitocin; see page 191), if magnesium sulfate is used, since the latter drug slows labor. Oxytocin also may be used to induce labor.

Mother's Reactions. During labor, she may feel

- Disappointment over the required interventions—induction, restriction to bed, and monitoring.
- Discomfort from the effects of medications, especially magnesium sulfate, which may make her twitch, sweat, and feel hot, flushed, and nervous. Blood-pressure medications may also have uncomfortable side effects—headaches, nausea, drowsiness, shortness of breath, and trouble urinating.

How You Can Help. You can sympathize with her, but help her focus on what she must do, for her own welfare and the baby's. Remind her of the comfort measures she still can use (see "When the Mother Must Labor in Bed," page 158).

Herpes Lesion

If the mother has or has ever had genital herpes, which causes sores to appear in the genital area, she should be sure to report this to her caregiver. If the virus is active when she goes into labor, the baby could contract the virus during vaginal birth. Herpes in the newborn is very serious; it frequently causes brain damage and death. If the mother has had herpes for a long time, the risk that a sore during labor could give the baby herpes is about 3 percent. The risk is higher if the mother has recently acquired herpes.

In an effort to prevent herpes outbreaks in late pregnancy, many caregivers offer anti-herpes medication (such as acyclovir) during the last weeks of pregnancy to all women who have ever had herpes sores. A woman who has not had an outbreak in years may reasonably refuse the medication, whereas a woman who has had one or more recent outbreaks may be wise to accept it.

If a woman has an outbreak at or near term, her caregiver will usually encourage her to take acyclovir, which can shorten the duration and severity of the outbreak (and perhaps provide protection for her baby). The caregiver may also offer to induce labor at a time when no sore is present.

Management During Labor if the Woman Has Herpes. At the hospital, the caregiver may

- Carefully inspect the genital area for the presence of a sore.
- Culture the mother's vaginal secretions for asymptomatic presence of the virus.
- Perform a cesarean to prevent the baby from coming into contact with a sore, if one is present.

If no sore is visible, but the culture later indicates that the herpes virus was present, the baby will be treated with an anti-herpes medication (acyclovir). Or the baby may be tested for herpes and treated only if the test indicates that the baby is infected.

Mother's Reactions. The mother will probably be disappointed, shocked, angry, or depressed when she learns she has an active herpes lesion, especially if she didn't expect it. If you were the source of her herpes, you may be the target of some of her anger. Expect her to need time, support, and perhaps counseling afterwards to deal with her disappointment over any changes in plans for the birth or any problems in the baby caused by the herpes.

Excessive Bleeding During Labor

Most bleeding comes from the site of the placenta. If the placenta begins to separate during labor, the woman will bleed; the

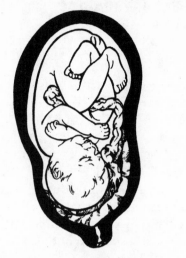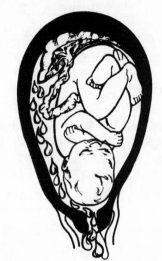

Left, *placenta previa;* right, *placental abruption.*

amount of visible bleeding and the seriousness of the problem depend on where and how extensive the separation is and whether bleeding is concealed, that is, blood does not flow out. If the placenta is very low in the uterus (this condition is called *placenta previa*), blood comes out of the vagina. If the placenta is high in the uterus when it begins to separate (this condition is called *placental abruption*), the uterus may become very firm between contractions, and the mother is in constant pain. Both mother and baby are in danger; this is potentially an acute emergency.

Management of Bleeding During Labor. This complication is managed in the following ways:

- If severe bleeding begins early in labor (or before labor begins), a cesarean delivery is probable. The mother may receive a general anesthetic if the blood loss is rapid; the anesthetic quickly puts the mother to sleep for the surgery.
- If bleeding begins late in labor, is not severe, and the fetus appears to be tolerating it, the doctor or midwife monitors the situation and waits. A vaginal birth may be possible.

Excessive Bleeding After Birth
(Postpartum Hemorrhage)

Some bleeding immediately after birth is normal; it comes from the area in the uterus where the placenta was attached. The uterus usually contracts vigorously after birth, causing the bleeding to subside. You may be surprised, though, at how much blood there seems to be even under normal circumstances. It usually amounts to a cup or so.

For a few weeks after birth a mother normally experiences a dwindling discharge, called lochia. The fluid is composed of blood and some of the tissue that lined the uterus during pregnancy. Lochia is like a longer-than-usual menstrual period.

Postpartum hemorrhage, or excessive bleeding after birth, usually occurs for one of three reasons: relaxation of the uterus, a retained placenta, or lacerations in the vagina or cervix. The loss of blood may cause the mother's blood pressure to drop; her skin may become clammy, and she may feel faint. To treat low blood pressure, the mother will be asked to lie flat, with her head low, and she will be given intravenous fluids, possibly containing a drug to raise her blood pressure.

Management of Bleeding After Birth. If the uterus relaxes after the birth, it leaves the blood vessels open at the placental site. When the uterus is made to contract, it will squeeze these vessels closed and the bleeding will stop.

- To make the uterus contract, the caregiver may vigorously massage the mother's uterus, inject drugs that contract the uterus—Pitocin or Methergine—into the mother's thigh, give Pitocin intravenously, or stimulate the mother's nipples to increase the body's secretion of oxytocin.
- If the placenta or parts of it are retained, the caregiver manually removes the placenta or the placental fragments. Since this procedure is very painful, it may be done while the mother is under anesthesia. If manual removal fails, surgery is required to clean out the uterus, tie off the large blood vessels, or, in very serious, life-threatening cases, to remove the uterus.
- If there are lacerations in the vagina or cervix, the lacerations are sutured.

The woman may receive blood transfusions if she loses a significant amount of blood.

How You Can Help. Do whatever you are told. A hemorrhage is an emergency, and quick action is essential. There is little time for explanations. If possible, remain with the mother and help her to cooperate in whatever she is asked to do.

(Please note: In the first few days after birth, the mother may notice that although she bleeds very little while lying down, when she stands up after a few hours in bed she suddenly may lose a lot of blood. This can be alarming, but it is probably due to the fact that blood collects in the vagina until gravity causes it to flow out. If heavy bleeding continues longer than a few minutes, however, or if the mother feels faint, call her caregiver or the hospital's maternity floor.)

The Breech Presentation

See page 160 for a discussion of management of the breech presentation.

Problems with Labor Progress

The caregiver or the nurse regularly observes and records the progress of labor. He or she performs vaginal exams to determine changes in the cervix and in the position and station of the fetus. The caregiver or nurse also observes the quality of the contractions (frequency, duration, and intensity) and the mother's reactions to them. Two situations that may signal problems are *very rapid progress* and *slow progress*.

Very Rapid Progress

When contractions are exceptionally efficient or unusually powerful, or when the cervix is exceptionally yielding, labor may progress rapidly. A fast labor may be extremely painful and frightening for the mother.

Main Concerns of the Caregiver. These are

- Getting the mother to the hospital in time (or in the case of a home birth, getting the caregiver to the home in time) to care for her adequately.
- How the fetus tolerates the powerful, frequent contractions.
- Damage to the mother's perineum during a rapid birth.
- The newborn's adjustment afterwards. Breathing problems and head trauma may be more likely as a result of this kind of birth.

Management of the Very Rapid Labor. This involves

- Supporting and reassuring the mother.
- Monitoring the response of the fetal heart to contractions and, possibly, using interventions (changing the mother's position, having her breathe oxygen) to improve oxygenation.
- Attempting to control the speed of delivery by coaching the mother not to bear down and by applying manual pressure against the rapidly emerging head.

How You Can Help. See "The Very Rapid Labor," pages 141 to 142.

Slow Progress in Active Labor

We generally expect dilation to speed up by the time the cervix has dilated to 4 or 5 centimeters. By this time the cervix is usually quite thin and ready to open more easily, even if it has taken many hours or even a day or two to reach this point (see "The Slow-to-Start Labor," page 137). Sometimes, though, dilation does not follow this expected pattern: It may be very slow (this is called *protracted labor*) or it may seem to stop for two or more hours (this is called *arrested labor*).

The reasons for a delay in the active phase are more likely to be serious than are the reasons for a slow prelabor or a slow latent phase. It is not always possible to determine why labor is delayed, nor is it possible to know just how serious the delay is until time has passed. The slow progress is not necessarily a problem in itself, but it may be a concern for the caregiver, who may begin to think that the labor should be hastened with medications.

Causes of Slow Progress in Labor. The delay may be due to one or a combination of causes:

- A poor fit between the baby's head and the mother's pelvis. This is sometimes called cephalo-pelvic disproportion, or CPD. *Cephalo* means head, and in the case of CPD the baby's head will not fit through the pelvis. The poor fit is more likely to be caused by the position of the baby's head than its size. If the baby is occiput posterior (OP, see page 44), or if her head is slightly tilted back with her chin up or to one side, her head will not fit as well as it will if she is in an occiput anterior (OA) position, with her chin on her chest and the top of her head centered on the cervix. Most babies in the OP position eventually rotate, causing labor to speed up. Some babies are born in the OP position, or with their heads tilted, although these births may take longer.
- Inadequate intensity of uterine contractions. They lose intensity, slow down, or become shorter in duration. Or they stay the same—too weak or too infrequent (or both).
- Exhaustion, dehydration, excessive fear, or tension in the mother.

Assessment of Delay in Labor. The caregiver tries to determine the cause(s) of the delay by assessing the contractions, the size and position of the baby, and the mother's physical and emotional state.

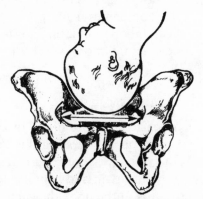

A poor fit between the baby's head and the mother's pelvis.

Many things can be done to speed a prolonged labor, and to support the woman undergoing it. Some of these things you and the mother can do; others must be done by the nurses and caregiver.

Patience is often the best management when a delay occurs. The caregiver patiently waits while the problem corrects itself, offers support and encouragement in the meantime, and watches the mother and fetus for signs of maternal problems or fetal distress. Although this usually results in resolution of the problem, the mother may have difficulty waiting if she is discouraged or tired. If she is being cared for by optimistic people, however, she will tolerate the wait amazingly well. While waiting, the mother can

- Eat easily digested, high-energy food (clear soups, toast with honey or jelly, yogurt, or sorbet) and drink fruit juices.
- Get into the shower or tub. This often relaxes her and reduces the emotional stress that may have slowed the labor.
- Benefit from additional labor support. A doula can be especially helpful under these circumstances. She can offer encouragement and remind the two of you of comfort measures and body positions that may make the slow progress tolerable. She can let you take a break for a snack, a nap, or some fresh air. If you do not have a doula, you might call a friend or relative to come. A fresh face often brings new energy.
- Refer to "Backache During Labor" (page 152) for a long list of things to do to turn a malpositioned baby, and to relieve the backache that accompanies many prolonged labors.
- Try the nonmedical labor-stimulating measures, especially walking and nipple stimulation (see "When Labor Must Start," page 147).

While waiting, the caregiver may

- Monitor the fetal heart rate more often, or continuously, to help determine if the fetus is tolerating the delay.
- Offer the woman a narcotic or regional anesthesia (an epidural block) to reduce pain and help her relax.
- Start intravenous fluids in the hope that improved hydration and some calories might reenergize the uterus.

If these measures do not result in better progress, the caregiver may

- Rupture the membranes (see page 187).
- Use intravenous oxytocin (Pitocin) to stimulate contractions (see "Induction or Augmentation of Labor," page 189). Speeding up labor is inappropriate if the problem seems to be a poor fit between the baby's head and the mother's pelvis, or the baby's malposition.
- Use forceps or a vacuum extractor (see pages 197 to 200) if the delay occurs in the birthing (second) stage.
- Recommend a cesarean delivery if there is no progress even with the passage of considerable time and after efforts have been made to correct the problem (see chapter 9).

How You Can Help. You can help the mother in these ways:

- Confer with the doula or nurse on ways to help the mother.
- Suggest the measures discussed here that may help the mother. She may not think of the bath, the positions, the labor-stimulating measures, or the medications.
- Since the mother may also be reluctant to do things to make her contractions more intense if she is already tired and discouraged, ask the nurse or midwife for help. She may be more able to encourage the mother to try.
- Be sure the mother recognizes that by trying these measures she may speed labor. Remind her that if she does not try them (or if they do not work), the next step will probably be Pitocin to speed labor and an epidural to ease her pain.
- Try to eat, and refresh yourself by washing your face and brushing your teeth, but do not leave the mother without someone else (a doula, a friend, or a relative) to help her.

Problems with the Fetus

Prolapsed Cord

On very rare occasions, the umbilical cord slips below the baby, into or through the cervix. This can occur before or during labor, and is a true obstetric emergency that can result in the baby's death if it is not promptly and correctly managed. The danger is this: The fetus depends on the cord for its oxygen supply; if the cord prolapses (slips into the vagina), it can be pinched by the fetus's head or body at the cervix. This obstructs blood flow through the cord and deprives the fetus of oxygen. The fetus can survive only a few minutes without oxygen.

Signs to Recognize. A prolapsed cord is most likely to happen if two conditions are present: (1) The fetus is in a breech presentation (buttocks or feet down), or the head is high or off the cervix; AND (2) the bag of waters breaks suddenly (or is ruptured by the caregiver), with a gush.

With this combination of circumstances, the cord may slip out around the fetal head or buttocks as the fluid escapes; then the fetus, who has been "floating," presses down upon the cord. It is extremely unlikely that a cord prolapse could occur if the fetus is already descended low in the pelvis and the head or buttocks are already pressing against the cervix. If the baby is low and against the cervix, the chance of the cord prolapsing is minuscule.

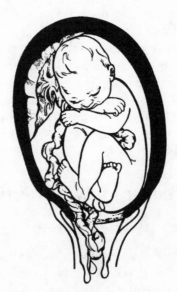

Prolapsed cord with a breech baby.

PROLAPSED CORD

CAUTION: In late pregnancy, the mother should ask her caregiver whether the baby is high and floating, low in the pelvis, or pressed against her cervix.

She should also ask, "If my bag of waters should break with my baby at this level of descent, should I be concerned about a prolapsed cord?" Then, if her caregiver says yes, she should do the following, with as much help from you as you can give her.

If she knows the fetus is high and if her bag of waters breaks with a gush of fluid

- She should call the caregiver and the hospital. If you can't drive her to the hospital, she should call 911 and tell them she is pregnant, her bag of waters broke, and she thinks she has a prolapsed cord. (See illustration on page 116.)
- With your help, she should get onto her hands and knees, and then drop her chest down to the floor or bed. This knee-chest position uses gravity to move the baby away from the cervix and off the cord.
- She should go immediately to the hospital. Before she stands up to walk quickly to the car, however, move the car close to the door of the house, adjust the seats, and leave the door open.
- She should ride in the back seat or in the ambulance in the knee-chest position.

Drive carefully, but waste no time. Drive to the hospital emergency entrance. Leave the mother in the car in the knee-chest position. Go in and tell the person on duty that your wife or friend is pregnant, her bag of waters broke, and you think she has a prolapsed cord. The mother should remain in the knee-chest position on a stretcher until a doctor or nurse can listen to the fetal heart rate. If the heart rate is normal, as it most likely will be, you can all try to relax and rejoice.

Management of a Prolapsed Cord. If the caregiver is present when the cord prolapses, he or she gets the mother into the knee-chest position and places a hand in the vagina to hold the baby off the cord. A cesarean section is performed as soon as possible. With this rapid action, the baby will probably be born in good health.

PROLAPSED CORD

How You Can Help. As scary as all this is, the odds of a prolapsed cord even if the baby is high or breech and the bag of waters breaks with a gush are low—perhaps 1 in 100. In the event of a cord prolapse, however, your actions and hers will be most important, since time and the mother's position are the crucial factors in the baby's well-being.

Cooperate with the hospital staff in whatever way possible.

Fetal Distress

Fetal distress means that the unborn baby is deprived of oxygen, and is showing signs of having to adjust physiologically. Although healthy babies have a remarkable ability to compensate for temporary oxygen deficits, brain damage can occur if oxygen deprivation is too severe and continues for too long, or if the baby already has a problem that reduces his ability to compensate.

How It Is Diagnosed. At present, the two best indicators of fetal distress are the fetal heart rate and blood chemistry. They are assessed in the following ways:

- A nurse or a midwife listens to the fetal heart rate with a fetal stethoscope or an ultrasound fetoscope at frequent intervals during labor. This requires that the nurse or midwife remain by the bedside much of the time.
- The caregiver monitors the fetal heart rate, as well as the strength of the mother's contractions, with an electronic fetal monitor (see page 180). A nurse observes the monitor tracings in the mother's room or, possibly, at the nurses' station.

Remember: If EFM indicates fetal distress, this does not necessarily mean that the baby is definitely in trouble. It may mean only that the baby is compensating for a temporary oxygen deficiency by slowing her heart rate to spare oxygen use. In other words, she may be in trouble, *or* she may be adjusting very well to the decrease in oxygen.

To find out if the baby really is in trouble, the caregiver needs to rely on more than EFM. Tests such as the fetal stimulation test (page 184) and fetal oxygen saturation monitoring (page

PROLAPSED CORD

180) can help reduce the likelihood of overdiagnosing and overtreating fetal distress. You might check ahead of time to see whether the mother's caregiver uses these other tests before performing cesareans for fetal distress.

Management of Fetal Distress. If monitoring indicates that the fetus may be in distress, the caregiver has these choices:

- Try to correct the fetal distress by having the mother breathe extra oxygen, which is carried via her bloodstream to the placenta and through the cord to the baby, and/or by having the mother change her position to relieve pressure on the umbilical cord, which may be causing the fetal distress.
- Call for further testing: Change from external to internal monitoring (the latter is more accurate), try the fetal stimulation test, or use fetal oxygenation saturation monitoring.
- If the fetal distress appears to be severe, immediately deliver the baby vaginally, with an episiotomy combined with the use of forceps or vacuum extraction, or by cesarean. The choice of delivery method depends on how close the mother is to giving birth.

Except for the fetal stimulation test, which takes only a few seconds or minutes, these corrective measures and tests take time, and depending on how the EFM tracing looks, the caregiver may be too anxious about the fetus's condition to wait for results. Because EFM, by itself, is sometimes inaccurate, cesareans are sometimes done that turn out to have been unnecessary.

Mother's Reactions. The mother is likely to react in these ways

- She will probably be very frightened and shocked when told that her baby shows signs of fetal distress.
- She will probably not question the caregiver's decisions under these circumstances.
- After the delivery, especially if it was sudden and frightening, the mother may have very mixed feelings: relief and joy that the baby is all right, confusion about all that has happened, and regrets or doubts about the cesarean and about her own behavior or decisions.

How You Can Help. You can help the mother in the following ways:

• Try to keep abreast of what is going on and what the staff is thinking.
• Ask questions. If the caregiver is worried that the baby is in danger, though, you do not want to keep him or her from doing what is necessary. You can ask for the quickly performed fetal stimulation test or fetal oxygenation saturation monitoring to confirm the diagnosis of fetal distress.
• Follow the suggestions given at the beginning of this chapter, page 202, keeping in mind that if the situation is urgent you will not have time for discussion.

Problems with the Newborn

The newborn baby is assessed immediately after birth. If all is normal, the baby is usually placed in the mother's arms for cuddling and suckling. If there are problems, the baby will probably go to the nursery for special care. It is beyond the scope of this book to cover newborn problems in detail, but I will list and discuss some fairly common problems that might arise shortly after birth.

If the baby has problems, take part in the decision making about appropriate care. The mother may be unable to think clearly right after the birth because of the excitement and the effects of drugs, exhaustion, or problems of her own. It falls upon you to become informed and to agree to the course of treatment.

If your baby must remain in the special-care nursery for several days or more, you will need to be your baby's advocate, despite your distress. When a baby is hospitalized, many caregivers (for example, pediatricians, neonatologists, other physician specialists, nurses, laboratory personnel, X-ray and ultrasound technicians, respiratory or physical therapists, and social workers) are usually involved. They come and go, each providing care and information according to their roles and responsibilities. Keeping track of everything can be most confusing and may seem next to impossible. Parents and their partners often feel helpless, depressed, and either distrustful of the baby's caregivers or resigned to accepting whatever they say. Good communication is the way to prevent these feelings of helplessness.

You should remain with the baby as much as possible. The baby needs someone who loves him close by, to hold him (if his condition permits), to stroke and talk to him, and to keep track of what is going on. When you need to leave, ask a relative or friend to stay with the baby. The point is to remain informed as the various professionals participate in the baby's care. Keep a written log of each visit, including the date, the time, the professional's name and specialty, the purpose of the visit, and a summary of any communication. Also write down your questions so you will not forget to ask them. Above all, you should know who is coordinating the baby's care, and how to reach that doctor or, when he or she is off duty, a substitute.

The mother should also remain with the baby as much as she is able. Try to be sure that there is a comfortable chair or bed for her, and that she has access to nourishing food. If the baby cannot breastfeed, the mother should be provided with a breast pump and instructions for using it. Pumped breast milk can usually be fed by bottle; if the baby cannot yet take a bottle, a stomach tube is used. Even if the mother is not planning to breastfeed, the pediatrician may ask her to provide her own milk until the baby can take formula well, since breast milk can help protect the baby from infection during this vulnerable time. Formula cannot do this.

Following are some immediate concerns about the baby.

Breathing

Breathing problems may be caused by fluid in the lungs, meconium aspiration (see "Suctioning the Nose and Mouth," page 277), narcotic drugs that were given to the mother inappropriately during labor (see chapter 8), infection, immature lungs, or other problems. A baby who is slow to breathe on her own, or who breathes very fast and grunts as she breathes, may need medications, intravenous feeding, an incubator, deep suctioning, resuscitation, mechanical assistance with breathing, extra oxygen, or other help.

Body Temperature

A baby whose body temperature drops below normal has to use up oxygen and energy trying to maintain it. It is important to keep the baby warm. (See "Warming Unit," page 281.)

Infection

A newborn sometimes acquires an infection while in the uterus or soon after birth. Depending on the organism causing it, the infection may be very serious (see "Group B Strep Screening," page 185). Prompt diagnosis and treatment with antibiotics or other medications, along with special care (intravenous feeding, an incubator, and close observation) in the nursery, are needed.

Since infection in a newborn can become very serious very quickly, painful interventions may be necessary. These may include spinal taps, bladder taps, heel sticks, scalp vein intravenous lines, nasogastric tubes, umbilical blood vessel tubes, and apnea monitors. Be sure that you are kept informed, and that there are good reasons to do any of these things to the baby.

Birth Trauma or Injury

Some babies are injured during the birth process, especially if the birth is difficult. A very rapid birth or a difficult forceps, vacuum, or cesarean delivery can cause bruises, a broken collar bone, or nerve damage. Although wise management reduces the chances of such injuries, they can occur even with the most skilled caregivers.

For some vulnerable babies (for example, premature babies, babies with birth defects, and babies with inherited or other preexisting problems), even the normal birth process is too much. Some very large babies also suffer, if great effort by the caregiver is required to deliver them. Vulnerable babies can usually, but not always, be identified before labor, and plans can be made in advance for their special care.

Sometimes, even with the best of care, a baby is unexpectedly born with serious problems requiring emergency treatment or long-term care. This possibility haunts parents and professionals alike, but also motivates attempts to develop better diagnostic and treatment methods.

Death of a Baby

On rare occasions a baby dies during or around the time of birth. Words cannot describe the shock and grief felt by the parents and their loved ones. Of course, nothing can bring the baby back to life, but memories can be created that will have great meaning as time passes.

As difficult as it is to think through the possibility that the baby could die, it is a good idea to find out the kinds of things that can be done to bring some positive meaning to such a tragedy. Please see page 29 for some suggestions. The reason for giving this some thought now is that decision making when one is grieving intensely is very difficult. Yet later parents may feel regret if they did not say goodbye in the way they would have chosen.

Many hospitals have sensitive and compassionate staff members who will do all they can to create a meaningful opportunity for parents to be alone with their baby. Please make a plan, then put it aside, with the peace of mind that you have it in case you need it. Now focus on a healthy outcome and a beautiful baby.

Drug Effects

If a baby is born with a drug in his system, the drug may noticeably affect his behavior. Depending on the drug, he may be sleepy, poor at sucking and breathing, lacking in muscle tone, irritable, jittery, jaundiced, or lacking in some reflex behaviors; or he may show other atypical signs. When the drug wears off, the baby behaves more normally. Sometimes other drugs (such as narcotic antagonists, which counteract some narcotic effects) or treatments (such as phototherapy, for jaundice) hasten the baby's recovery.

Low Blood Sugar

Low blood sugar is rather common in (1) babies of diabetic mothers, (2) very large babies, (3) babies whose mothers received large amounts of intravenous solutions of dextrose in water during labor, (4) babies born after prolonged labors, and (5) babies born under certain other conditions. The diagnosis of low blood sugar is made by drawing blood from the baby's heel and analyzing it. Treatment usually consists of giving the baby some glucose water, formula, or colostrum and rechecking blood sugar levels. The problem usually resolves itself quickly.

Jaundice

If the baby's skin or the whites of her eyes become yellowish, the baby is jaundiced. Usually harmless, *physiologic jaundice* is caused by high levels of bilirubin, a yellow pigment that results when red blood cells break down as part of their normal life cycle. Physiologic jaundice goes away on its own, usually in a few days, but high levels of bilirubin in some vulnerable babies may cause brain damage. Premature babies, babies who had particular difficulties during birth, and those with blood types incompatible with their mothers' are more vulnerable to brain damage from high bilirubin levels.

Jaundice is diagnosed by measuring bilirubin in the baby's blood, a sample of which is taken through a heel stick. Further tests of blood type, liver function, and bowel function help determine the cause of jaundice.

Jaundice is treated with phototherapy, which consists of keeping the baby under special bright lights almost constantly for a few days. Light breaks down (photo-oxidizes) bilirubin in the blood vessels of the baby's skin and thus lowers bilirubin levels. Portable phototherapy lights are available for treatment at home, as are blankets containing fiberoptic light filaments; one of these blankets can be wrapped around or placed under the baby. Prolonged exposure to indirect sunlight (through a window) is as effective, though not as reliable, as artificial light. Frequent nursing (more than eight times per day) also helps relieve jaundice.

If the bilirubin levels are very high or if the baby is premature, jaundice is more serious, and a complete exchange transfusion of the baby's blood may be done.

Prematurity or Low Birth Weight

The premature infant (born before 37 weeks' gestation) or the low-birth-weight infant (weighing less than 5½ pounds) is more susceptible to all the newborn problems described here than is the full-term, average-sized baby. Premature babies are therefore watched more closely and receive more aggressive treatment. As they approach average size and weight their vulnerability to problems decreases.

After It Is All Over

I have discussed numerous problems that can arise in both mother and child during labor and the early postpartum period. Each of these presents a challenge to all of you—to the mother, to the caregiver, to the baby, and to you, the birth partner.

Each problem takes an emotional toll requiring quick acceptance of a change in plans and expectations, often without a complete understanding of the situation. At the time, of course, you do what has to be done, even if you are almost in a state of shock. But afterwards, as you and the mother look back over the events, the feelings hit. Even if both the mother and the baby have come through it alive and healthy, the emotional impact can be great. Unanswered questions and feelings of guilt, anger, or disappointment may arise, especially if it all happened too quickly for either or both of you to grasp, or if the mother or the baby was treated unkindly or disrespectfully.

It may take time, especially for the mother, to come to terms with her unrealized expectations. Your patience and acceptance of what is, in reality, a grieving process will help. A conference with the mother's caregiver may help to fill gaps in understanding of the events and answer questions. Sometimes consulting with a childbirth educator or counselor helps either or both of you to sort out your feelings and gain a healthy perspective on a physically or emotionally traumatic birth experience. Please see page 263, "Your Role During Cesarean Birth," for further discussion of emotional reactions following a difficult birth.

In the end, with the birth behind her, let us hope that the mother recognizes the courage and grace she displayed as she dealt with the unexpected challenges posed by a problem labor.

8

Medications for Pain During Labor

Next to the health of mother and baby, the major concern of the caregiver, the birth partner, and the mother herself is the mother's comfort during labor. Although the pain of labor is very intense, it does not have to be overwhelming. There is much the mother can do to keep it manageable. She can learn and rehearse many effective comfort measures in childbirth classes (see "Comfort Measures for Labor," page 95). It is essential for you to help her carry them out; labor is simply too demanding for her to use all she has learned without help.

In addition to these comfort measures, drugs can be used to relieve labor pain. To a great extent drugs are optional; the mother can decide whether and when to use them. Because they are readily available, and because they can have profound effects, the mother should learn about the available drugs in advance and decide how she feels about using them during labor. You should also be prepared. Do your attitudes toward pain medications match the mother's? Can you agree? Find out in advance how she feels about pain medications, and plan to support her in accomplishing what she wants.

It may seem somewhat foolish for a woman to plan her use of pain medications in advance, since she has no idea how much pain she will feel or how she will react. But she really does not have to know these things to make a good decision ahead of time. Using the information in this chapter, you and the mother can make a plan that will guide you both as you encounter the pain of labor together.

Management of Normal Labor Without Pain Medications

The pain of normal labor, though severe, can be successfully managed without the use of pain medications if

- *The mother wants to avoid pain medications.* Obviously, she is more likely to avoid medications if she wants to. She decides just how important it is to her.
- *She has prepared herself for childbirth.* She needs to know alternatives to medications: comfort measures such as relaxation, patterned breathing, movement, positions, and massage. It helps if the two of you have rehearsed these together. She will also cope better is she has access to such aids as a bath, a shower, a rocking chair, a birth ball, hot packs, cold packs, a squatting bar, and music. If she will be giving birth in a hospital that does not provide these aids, you might bring some of them. (See "Comfort Measures for Labor," page 95.)
- *She has emotional support and assistance.* She needs competent, caring support from you—someone who loves her, who knows her well, who wants to share the birth, and who wants to help her accomplish her wishes.

    The continuous help of a doula improves a woman's chances of using less pain medication or avoiding it altogether, if that is what she wants. The doula accomplishes this with encouragement, reassurance, information, and guidance in the use of techniques that lessen pain and help labor progress. A doula brings confidence, empathy, experience, and understanding to a birth.

The mother also needs the support of the professional staff. A woman in labor is vulnerable to both positive and negative suggestions, especially from the experts—nurses, midwives, and physicians. If they believe in her and encourage her, she is more likely to carry on; if they pity, ignore, or discourage her, she is more likely to give up.

- *She has a reasonably normal labor.* This is partly a matter of luck. It must be a labor that does not include problems requiring many painful interventions, one that does not thoroughly exhaust and discourage her. This does not mean labor has to be short or painless. If the first three conditions are present, a woman can handle a long, hard labor very well without pain medications.

If the mother prefers a medication-free labor, prepare yourself well for an active support role.

What You Need to Know about Pain Medications

To make an informed decision about pain medications, you and the mother both need some information: What is the drug? How does it work? How effective is it in relieving pain? What other effects does it have—on the mother, on the progress of labor, on the fetus, and on the newborn? What precautions or added interventions are needed to ensure safety? Do not wait until the mother is in labor to get this information. When she is in pain and asking for medication, it is too late to try to learn all about the drugs.

Remember that, although various drugs are available, effective, and widely used in labor, they involve a tradeoff: the mother gets pain relief, but she or the fetus may experience unwanted side effects—directly, from the drug itself, or indirectly, through potential problems such as restriction of the mother's activity or the need for other interventions. Long-term effects on the baby of drugs used judiciously in labor have not been established. There may be no harm, or, in some cases, there may be subtle long-term effects. This is a subject of great debate in the medical literature, and it is unlikely to be settled in the near future.

For these reasons I advocate learning about the nondrug methods of pain relief (see "Comfort Measures for Labor," page 95) and seeking a birth place that has the amenities (bathtub, shower, squatting bar, birthing bed, places to walk, rocking chair) that enhance a laboring woman's comfort. You may bring your own music, hot or cold packs, and birth ball (see page 121) if the hospital or birth center doesn't have one.

These nondrug methods are very helpful, and by using them for at least part of the labor the mother can comfortably postpone her use of pain medications and reduce the total amount of medications she receives. By doing so, she lessens the likelihood of undesirable effects and the need for additional interventions.

Many women find these nondrug methods sufficient to keep their pain at a level at which they can cope throughout the labor. Afterward, the absence of drug side effects and the ability to get up and move freely immediately after the birth contribute to a feeling that the rewards are worth the pain.

Preparing to deal with labor pain through nondrug methods, however, is time consuming, and going through labor without drugs can be a challenge. And if labor is exhausting or complicated, the benefits of pain medications will outweigh the potential risks. Effective methods of pain medication, most notably the epidural, are widely available in hospitals. Many women choose the epidural as an easy way to get through labor.

As you both learn more about pain medication, you will be able to help the mother make informed choices. To begin our discussion of pain medications, here are several definitions.

- *Analgesia.* Reduction of pain. Analgesics are drugs that relieve pain.
- *Anesthesia.* Loss of sensation, including pain sensation. Anesthetics are drugs that take away feeling.
- *Systemic.* Taken up by the bloodstream, affecting the entire body, and reaching the baby in similar concentrations.
- *Regional.* Affecting an area of the body that is supplied by specific spinal nerves.
- *Regional anesthetic or analgesic.* A pain medication injected near nerve roots in the spine to block or decrease awareness of pain in the area supplied by those spinal nerves.
- *Local.* Affecting specific tissues—in childbirth, the cervix,

vagina, and perineum. A local anesthetic blocks the function of nerve endings only in these tissues.

- *General anesthesia.* Complete loss of consciousness caused by a systemic medication, a *general anesthetic.*

When pain medications are used, several factors influence the degree and area of pain relief and the severity of side effects:

- The choice of medication—a narcotic or narcotic-like drug, a sedative, a tranquilizer, an anesthetic gas, an injected anesthetic, an amnesiac.
- The total dose—the concentration of the drug, the volume of each dose, and the number of doses.
- The route of administration—injection into a muscle, a vein, the cervix or vaginal wall; inhalation into the lungs; injection into the epidural or spinal (intrathecal) space; swallowing into the stomach.
- Individual characteristics of the mother—her weight, her sensitivity to medications, her clotting ability, her anatomic variations, her physical condition, the duration of her pregnancy, and her overall health.

How Pain Is Relieved by Medications

Medications reduce pain by altering some part of the nervous system, the system that makes it possible to recognize, interpret, and react to pain.

Labor pain originates with pressure, stretching, or compression involving tissues in the uterus, vagina, or pelvic joints. Contractions of the uterus, dilation of the cervix, and the baby's movement through the pelvis create the pain. Nerve endings in these tissues are stimulated to send pain impulses over nerve fibers to the spinal cord and brain.

The transmission of the pain signals can be modified anywhere along this pathway—in the nerve endings, in the nerve roots (which are located where the nerves leave the spine); in the spinal cord, or in the brain.

This is how various pain medications work:

- Local anesthetics prevent nerve endings from sending the pain impulses over the nerve fibers to the spine and brain.

- Epidural and spinal medications interrupt the transmission of pain signals in the nerve fibers just before or as they enter the spinal cord.
- Systemic medications (such as narcotics) act in the brain to reduce recognition of pain or reactions to it.

The rest of this chapter presents specific information about the various medications used during labor. Use these pages as a guide for making decisions and for seeking further information. The drugs are grouped according to general characteristics (there are subtle differences, which are not described here, among the drugs in each group). The chart "When Can Pain Medication Be Used?," page 252, lists these groups of drugs and indicates at which stages of labor they are most safely given and when their effects will ideally have worn off. Use this quick guide and the more detailed information in this chapter as general background for your discussions about pain medications with the mother and her caregiver. When you both have read through the chapter, you will be ready to use the "Pain Medications Preference Scale," on pages 249 to 251, as a tool in your decision making.

Systemic Drugs

Drugs that affect the whole body—the entire system—are called *systemic drugs*. Systemic analgesics (pain-relieving drugs) use the bloodstream to transport the medication to the brain, where the drug exerts its pain-relieving effect. Systemic drugs can be given in several forms: as pills, as gases to inhale, or as injections—into the skin or muscle, or directly into the vein.

Systemic drugs circulate not only to the mother's brain but throughout her body; they also cross the placenta to the baby. Because their effects on the baby after birth may be profound, these drugs must be given early enough in the labor to allow time for them to wear off before birth. If a systemic drug has not worn off sufficiently by the time of birth, another drug, such as a narcotic antagonist, is given to counteract the unwanted effects of the original drug.

Even when the timing is appropriate, some of a drug (or its metabolic by-products) almost certainly remains in the baby's bloodstream after birth and subtly alters his behavior and reflexes for a few days following. How severely medication affects the baby depends on his health and maturity, the choice of drug, the size and number of doses given, and the times they are given during labor. The healthier the baby, the smaller the amount of medication used, and the greater the time between its administration and the birth, the less pronounced the effects will be on the baby.

There are three categories of systemic pain medications that may be given during prelabor or during the dilation (first) stage: tranquilizers, sedatives, and narcotics (see the table on page 252). Another group of systemic medications, general anesthetics, are occasionally used during the dilation or birthing (second) stage. General anesthetics are discussed as a separate category on page 232.

Regional Analgesia and Anesthesia (Epidural and Spinal)

Of all the pain-relieving medications, regional anesthetics and analgesics provide the most effective pain relief, use the smallest amount of drug, and have the least effects on the mother's mental state and on the baby's well-being. Depending on the dosage, these drugs cause partial to complete numbness and reduction or loss of control over movement and muscle strength, body temperature, blood pressure, ability to urinate, and other functions.

Regional blocks may be used for both vaginal and cesarean deliveries. They do not alter the mother's consciousness, unless narcotics, which cause some grogginess, are given with the anesthetic. Administration of these drugs requires a high degree of skill, and is therefore done only by specialists—anesthesiologists or specially trained nurse-anesthetists. Regional blocks are the most costly of all obstetric pain-relieving techniques.

Either the spinal or the epidural block can be given as a single injection or, for more prolonged anesthesia, via a catheter (a thin tube) inserted and left in place. With a catheter, the medication can be administered either as a continuous drip or, at the push of a button, in patient-controlled doses. A spinal is usually given as a single injection; the effects last a few hours.

Both the spinal and the epidural blocks are given in the *lumbar spine*, in the low back. The spinal is given through the *dura* and into the *dural space*. The dura is the membrane that surrounds the spinal cord and the spinal nerves and contains the spinal fluid; the dural space is the space within the dura. The epidural block is also given in the lumbar spine, but in the *epidural space*, just outside the dura.

General Characteristics of Regional and Local Anesthesia. The drugs used for regional and local blocks are sometimes referred to as "caine" drugs; common examples are Carbocaine, Marcaine, Xylocaine, Nesacaine, and Ropivacaine. These drugs are quite similar in their effects on the mother, on the labor, and on the baby. Subtle differences in their biochemical makeup, however, affect the way they act in the body and the duration of their effects. The mother's caregiver and her anesthesiologist usually select the specific drug to be used. The mother should be sure to inform the anesthesiologist if she has a sensitivity or allergy to any drug.

Narcotics, such as morphine, fentanyl, and sufentanil, are often given in spinals and epidurals, either alone or in combination with the "caine" anesthetics.

Narcotics take effect more quickly than the caine drugs and interfere less with a woman's use of her legs. If narcotics are given alone in early labor, the mother may be able to walk a bit with your help. But she may not be very steady on her feet, so do not be out of arm's reach. A caine drug may be added in active labor, when the pain becomes more intense.

Narcotics can cause side effects on the mother, and may affect the baby, too. In many women these drugs cause grogginess, itching, and nausea. Fentanyl and sufentanil, because of their biochemical properties, cross more easily to the baby than the caine drugs. The effects on the newborn have not been studied.

Epidural and spinal narcotics are becoming popular for pain relief after a cesarean. A dose given before the mother leaves the operating room provides very good pain relief for about 24 hours, after which she is offered other pain medications.

In general, the desired effect of the drugs is loss of pain sensation in the area anesthetized. Reducing her pain relaxes the mother and may result in more rapid dilation of the cervix, especially in a prolonged, exhausting labor. Other possible effects (depending on the area injected, the total dosage, and the choice of drug) include the following:

• *On the mother:* Reduced use of legs; a drop in blood pressure; a temporary slowing of labor; fever (her temperature may increase with the duration of the epidural); a loss or reduction of the bearing-down reflex in the second (birthing) stage; a need for vacuum extraction or a forceps delivery; a spinal headache, and, rarely, a toxic reaction to the drug.
• *On the fetus:* Temporary changes in the heart rate caused by lower maternal blood pressure; fever; a rapid heart rate due to fever.
• *On newborn:* (depending on the amount of the drug in the baby's blood): Subtle changes in suckling ability; decreased attentiveness; increased fussiness. These effects seem to last for only a few days.

Technique for Giving a Regional Block. There are many similarities among the techniques for administering the various regional blocks. The general procedure is described here. Please refer to the table "Pain Medications and Their Effects," page 238, for specific information about each type of block.

Regional blocks numb or reduce sensation in a large portion of the mother's body—between the top of her uterus and her feet. The area affected can be controlled by the amount and concentration of the drug given and by the placement of the injection. For example, the mother may be able to move her legs while remaining numb in her trunk. This is the procedure:

1. Before receiving the anesthetic, the mother is given intravenous (IV) fluids to reduce the chance that her blood pressure will drop.
2. The mother lies on her side or sits up and leans forward. An anesthesiologist scrubs the area where the injection will be given, numbs the skin with a local anesthetic, and then injects a small amount of anesthetic between the vertebrae of her low back (lumbar spine), into the epidural or dural space (see the

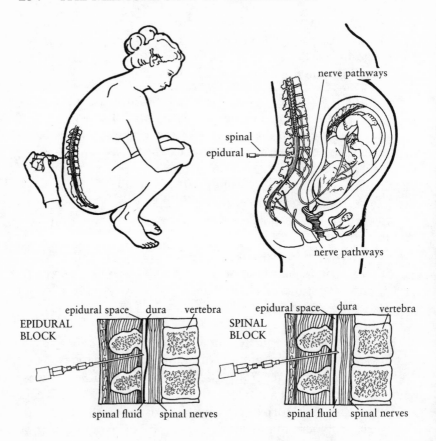

Regional anesthesia. Above left: *As the mother lies on her side, the anesthesiologist injects the anesthetic.* Above right: *The sites of injection for regional blocks.* Below: *These detailed drawings illustrate the placement of the needle for an epidural block* (left) *and a spinal block* (right).

illustrations). The anesthesiologist checks to make sure that the needle is placed correctly.

3. A full dose is given. Within minutes the mother begins to feel the effects. She is soon numb in the desired area.

4. Sometimes pain relief is uneven or spotty, and it takes some adjustment (changing the mother's position, injecting more doses) before the pain relief is adequate.

5. A thin plastic tube (a catheter) can be left in her back so that the medicine may drip in steadily or the mother may add some, by pushing a button, if she desires.

6. The mother's blood pressure and pulse are checked frequently.

Before choosing an epidural or spinal for pain relief during labor, consider that a rather long time may pass from when the decision is made to use anesthesia until the mother is comfortable. The time involved in preparing the mother, waiting for the anesthesiologist to arrive, administering the drug, and allowing the medication to take effect adds up to 30 to 60 minutes or more. This is a difficult time for the mother; she has decided she does not want to cope any more, and yet she still has to. She may find it harder than ever to wait for the anesthetic to be given and to take effect. You will have to continue encouraging her in breathing, attention focusing, and distraction until she gets relief from the pain. Sometimes, a mother is progressing so fast in labor that she no longer needs the extra pain relief by the time it takes effect. She may be pushing her baby out by then!

Local Anesthesia

The local blocks are given via injection. There are three major local blocks: the paracervical, the pudendal, and the perineal. The paracervical block numbs the cervix; the pudendal block numbs the birth canal, or the vagina; and the perineal block numbs the perineum. The perineal is the one usually called a "local."

Technique for Giving Local Anesthesia. Local blocks numb smaller portions of the mother's body than do regional blocks. Giving local anesthetics does not require the skills of an anesthesiologist, because these blocks are easier to administer. The caregiver draws the anesthetic into a syringe and injects it into the appropriate sites within or near the vagina. For details about each type of block, see the table "Pain Medications and Their Effects" (page 238).

Local blocks require larger doses of medication and provide less pain relief than do regional blocks. Also, with a local block more medication enters the mother's circulation; the drug may thus affect the fetus and the newborn more profoundly than it would if administered in a regional block. Because of these disadvantages, the paracervical block has almost disappeared from use in many areas of North America, and the pudendal block now tends to be reserved for late second-stage forceps deliveries. The perineal block, or "local," is given either shortly before delivery for an episiotomy, or immediately after delivery for stitching. If the anesthetic is administered close to delivery, the fetus may receive less of the drug and be less affected.

General Analgesia and Anesthesia

General anesthetics are systemic drugs (affecting the whole body). Given in the form of a gas to be inhaled through a mask, they rapidly enter the bloodstream via the lungs. They circulate to the brain, where they quickly relieve or abolish the awareness of pain and cause loss of consciousness. Though easy and quick to administer, general anesthetics carry the potential risk that the unconscious woman may vomit and inhale her vomitus, which causes pneumonia. Although anesthesiologists are trained to prevent such a complication, regional anesthesia is safer and therefore generally preferred. But general anesthesia might be used today in the following circumstances:

- When life-threatening complications to the mother (such as hemorrhage) or baby (such as a prolapsed cord) require a cesarean or other surgery to be performed within minutes.
- When a regional block cannot be performed because of illness or anatomical anomalies in the woman.
- When an unexpected cesarean must be performed in a rural hospital that does not have an anesthesiologist on duty around the clock.
- When the woman expressed a strong desire to be unconscious for the birth.

See the table "Pain Medications and Their Effects" (pages 238 to 247) for an explanation of the effects of different concentrations of inhaled gases.

Deciding Whether to Use
Pain Medications During Labor

It is important for you to know the mother's desires regarding her use of pain medications in labor, and to explore with her how you yourself feel about her using them. Many birth partners have strong personal feelings on the subject. Some believe deeply that natural childbirth is preferable; others believe that natural childbirth is unnecessary suffering and encourage the use of medications. The most important thing is for both of you to share your feelings in advance and then prepare together as described here. Use the "Pain Medications Preference Scale," pages 249 to 251, to thoroughly explore the way you both feel.

When you both have learned about the demands and joys of childbirth, and about the medical and nonmedical methods to manage pain, it is time to come up with a plan regarding the use of pain medication that meets the laboring woman's wishes. Both of you should examine your personal feelings about birth, pain, and the support the mother needs. How much help can she realistically expect from you? How do you honestly feel about taking on the role of the birth partner? Go through the list of questions headed "How Will You Feel" (page 11) to a ssess your reactions to some of the realities of labor.

The "Pain Medications Preference Scale" (PMPS) offers her a systematic and realistic way to think about her preferred approach to pain relief and the kind of help she will need from you and others. You too should go through the PMPS, to see if the two of you agree in your feelings about her use of pain medications.

Of course, no one knows in advance how long or painful a woman's labor will be or whether there will be complications. A flexible approach is the only sensible one. The PMPS takes this into account by including a variety of possibilities.

After thoughtful consideration of these unknowns, her desires—as she expresses them with the PMPS before labor—are a good predictor of whether or not she will use pain medications. They are also a most helpful guide to all who will be helping her.

PAIN MEDICATIONS AND THEIR EFFECTS

Drug Names, and How and Where Given	Desired Effects	Other Possible Effects	Precautions and Procedures for Safe Use
SYSTEMIC MEDICATIONS			
Morphine • Given by injection into muscle or vein. • Given in pre- or early labor.	• Therapeutic rest. • Temporary stop to non-productive contractions. • Feeling of well-being.	*Mother:* Drop in blood pressure, dizziness, restlessness or excessive sedation, confusion, nausea and vomiting, urinary retention, respiratory depression. *Fetus:* Hypoxia, drop in fetal heart rate, decreased movement. *Baby:* Heart rate changes, respiratory depression, need for resuscitation, depression of suckling and other reflexes.	Restriction to bed, continuous fetal monitoring, oxygen for the mother or baby, administration of nalaxone (drug to reverse side effects), timing of dosage to avoid the greatest risks to the baby.
Sedatives/Barbiturates pentobarbital (Nembutal), secobarbital (Seconal) • Given by injection or pill. • Used during the first stage before 4 cm dilation to allow effects on the baby to diminish before birth.	• Sleepiness, relaxation. • Possible slowing of unproductive contractions. • Reduction in anxiety and tension.	*Mother:* Increased perception of pain, dizziness, confusion, restlessness, excitement, disorientation, nausea, nightmares after use; depressed respiration. *Fetus:* Heart-rate changes. *Baby:* Poor suckling, breathing problems, decreased alertness, decreased attention span for 2 to 4 days.	Oxygen for the mother or baby; resuscitation equipment for the baby; avoidance of concurrent use of narcotics.

238

Tranquilizers	• Drowsiness, relaxation.	*Mother:* Dizziness, confusion, dry mouth, blood-pressure and heart-rate changes. Versed causes amnesia of birth and the first hours with the baby. *Fetus:* Heart-rate changes. *Baby:* Problems with breathing, temperature, and nursing; jaundice; lack of muscle tone and alertness.	Versed and Valium are considered too risky to the fetus and newborn to be used during labor. They are reserved for cesarean deliveries, and then used in small doses.
promethazine (Phenergan), promazine (Sparine), hydroxyzine (Vistaril), midazolam (Versed), diazepam (Valium)	• Reduction in tension, anxiety, nausea, and vomiting.		
	• Reduction of side effects of some narcotics.		
• Given by injection or pill.	• Possible acceleration of labor in a tense, exhausted woman.		
• Used during the first stage before 7 cm dilation.			
• May be used for cesarean delivery for profound tranquilizing effects.			
Narcotic and Narcotic-like Analgesics	• Partial relief of pain, relaxation.	*Mother:* Nausea, dizziness, "high" or groggy feeling, hallucinations, low heart rate and blood pressure, confusion, depressed respiration, temporary slowing of labor. *Fetus:* Heart-rate changes, decreased movement. *Baby:* Heart-rate changes; depressed respiration at birth, which may require resuscitation; poor suckling; depression of other reflexes.	Oxygen for the mother or baby; nalaxone (a narcotic antagonist) for the mother or baby to counter depressive effects; effort to predict the time of birth to avoid giving the drug when the risks to the baby are greatest.
meperidine (demerol), nalbuphine (Nubain), fentanyl (Sublimaze), butorphanol (Stadol), pentazocine (Talwin)	• Halting, slowing, or speeding of contractions, depending on the amount, timing, and drug used.		
• Given by injection or IV.			
• Used during first stage until 7 cm dilation.			

Continued on next page

Drug Names, and How and Where Given	Desired Effects	Other Possible Effects	Precautions and Procedures for Safe Use
Narcotic Antagonist naloxone (Narcan) • May be given to the mother or baby after birth, if needed, to reverse the side effects of a narcotic. • Given by injection into the muscle or vein.	• Reversal of some effects of narcotics on mother or baby, such as hallucinations, depressed respiration, low blood pressure and heart rate, diminished newborn reflexes and poor suckling.	*Mother:* Nausea, vomiting, sweating, shivering, restlessness, increased heart rate, return of pain, high blood pressure, heart arrythmias, pulmonary edema (rarely), tremors. *Fetus:* Increased activity, improved heart rate *Baby:* No effects observed when the drug is used to reverse respiratory depression in the newborn.	Possible supplemental doses after 30 to 45 minutes, or the effects of the narcotic may return.
Inhalation Analgesia nitrous oxide gas and oxygen (Entonox). • Self-administered by mother. • Given late in the first stage, in the second stage, and occasionally in the third stage.	• Loss of pain awareness and consciousness for about a minute, followed by quick recovery.	*Mother:* Temporary difficulty in rational thought and in bearing down during birthing contractions. *Fetus:* Transient effect. *Baby:* Little effect on newborn after the mother self-administers the drug; long-term effects unknown.	The mother begins inhaling nitrous oxide about 30 seconds before the onset of a contraction, to erase pain and consciousness through the peak. If she waits until the contraction begins before inhaling the gas, relief comes only after the contraction has peaked.

REGIONAL ANESTHESIA

Standard Lumbar Epidural
mepivacaine (Carbocaine),
chloroprocaine (Nesacaine),
bupivacaine (Marcaine),
Lidocaine (Xylocaine),
Ropivacaine (Naropin)

- Injected into a catheter
placed in the epidural space
outside the spinal canal; may
be given as a continuous
drip.
- Given before 8 cm dilation,
or later if labor is slow or arrested.

- Loss of pain sensation from
abdomen to toes.
- Relaxation as pain is
relieved.
- Sleep for an exhausted
mother.

Mother: Inability to move the
lower half of her body; toxic
reaction (rare); after four
hours, fever that increases with
the duration of the epidural;
decrease in blood pressure;
slowing of labor; reduced
urge and ability to push;
spinal headache if the needle
is inadvertently injected into
the dural space; increased
chance of forceps, vacuum
extractor, or cesarean delivery.
Fetus: Heart-rate changes and
lack of oxygen, caused by low
maternal blood pressure and
fever.
Baby: Subtle changes in
reflexes, including suckling
and breathing; fussiness.

Mother: Restriction to bed,
frequent checks of blood pressure and blood oxygenation,
withholding of food and drink,
intravenous fluids, bladder
catheter, oxygen mask, continuous electronic fetal monitoring, oxytocin to augment
contractions, forceps or
vacuum extractor, episiotomy,
increased chance of cesarean.
Baby: Blood, urine, or spinal-
fluid cultures to detect infection, antibiotics, and 48 hours
in a special-care nursery for
observation if the mother had
a fever in labor.

Continued on next page

241

PAIN MEDICATIONS AND THEIR EFFECTS—*Continued*

Drug Names, and How and Where Given	Desired Effects	Other Possible Effects	Precautions and Procedures for Safe Use
Segmental Lumbar Epidural ("light and late") mepivacaine (Carbocaine), chloroprocaine (Nesacaine), bupivacaine (Marcaine), lidocaine (Xylocaine), ropivacaine (Naropin), mixed with low doses of narcotics (fentanyl or sufentanil). • A lower concentration of anesthetic than for a standard epidural is injected into the epidural space outside the spinal canal. • Given as a continuous drip into a catheter, or self-administered. Self-administration generally reduces the amount of medication and its side effects. • Given in the first stage, usually after 5 cm dilation.	• Loss of pain sensation in the trunk, without total loss of movement and sensation in the perineum and legs. • Relaxation as pain is relieved. • Sleep for an exhausted mother.	*Mother* (most of these are less likely with a "light and late" than with a standard lumbar epidural): After four hours, fever that increases with the duration of the epidural; decrease in blood pressure; slowing of labor; reduced urge and ability to push; spinal headache if the needle is inadvertently injected into the dural space; increased chance of forceps, vacuum extractor, or cesarean delivery. *Fetus:* Heart-rate changes and lack of oxygen, caused by low maternal blood pressure and fever. *Baby:* Subtle changes in reflexes, including suckling and breathing; fussiness.	*Mother:* Restriction to bed, frequent checks of blood pressure and blood oxygenation, withholding of food and drink, intravenous fluids, bladder catheter, oxygen mask, continuous electronic fetal monitoring, oxytocin to augment contractions, forceps or vacuum extractor, episiotomy, increased chance of cesarean. *Baby:* Blood, urine, or spinal-fluid cultures to detect infection, antibiotics, and 48 hours in a special-care nursery for observation if the mother had a fever in labor.

Type of Medication	Benefits	Possible Side Effects	Medical Interventions
Epidural Narcotics ("Walking Epidural") and Spinal (Intrathecal) Narcotics meperidine (Demerol), morphine (Duramorph), fentanyl (Sublimaze), sufentanil (Sufenta) • Epidural: Given by injection or continuous drip into the epidural space outside the spinal canal. • Spinal: Given as an injection into the dural space in the spinal canal. • Used during the first stage or after a cesarean delivery.	• Long-term pain relief with no change in mental state. • Retention of enough muscle function in the legs that the woman can often stand and walk with help, and move freely in bed.	*Mother:* Nausea, vomiting, urine retention, itching, spinal headache (caused by leaking of spinal fluid); "breakthrough" pain at 6 to 8 cm dilation if only narcotics are used. *Fetus:* Heart-rate changes (these occur less frequently with epidural than with IV narcotics). *Baby:* Narcotics are absorbed by the baby, but the effects are unknown.	Intravenous fluids and oxytocin; narcotic antagonist to control side effects; bladder catheter; blood patch (some of the mother's blood is injected into the dura to form a clot to stop leaking of spinal fluid and relieve a spinal headache); continuous fetal monitoring; increased chance of forceps or vacuum extractor delivery and episiotomy.
Spinal Block mepivacaine (Carbocaine), chloroprocaine (Nesacaine), bupivacaine (Marcaine), lidocaine (Xylocaine) • Usually given as a single injection into the dural space in the spine. • Given any time before or during labor for a planned or unplanned cesarean. • Not used for vaginal births today.	• Easier to administer than an epidural block. • More rapid onset of pain relief than with an epidural. • Loss of pain, other sensations, and movement from waist to toes for two to three hours after injection, with no mental effects. • Relaxation and rest as pain is relieved.	*Mother:* Toxic reaction (rare); decrease in blood pressure; spinal headache (caused by leaking of spinal fluid); impaired breathing, requiring artificial ventilation, if the level of anesthesia rises high enough to affect the muscles in the chest. *Fetus:* Heart-rate changes, caused by low maternal blood pressure. *Baby:* Subtle changes in reflexes, including suckling and breathing; lack of attentiveness and muscle tone; fussiness.	Frequent checks of blood pressure and blood oxygenation, electrocardiogram, intravenous fluids, bladder catheter, oxygen mask, artificial ventilation, continuous fetal monitoring until cesarean begins, blood patch (see "Epidural and Spinal Narcotics," above).

Continued on next page

PAIN MEDICATIONS AND THEIR EFFECTS—*Continued*

Drug Names, and How and Where Given	Desired Effects	Other Possible Effects	Precautions and Procedures for Safe Use
Combined Spinal/Epidural (CSE) fentanyl (Sublimaze) or sufentanil (Sufenta) plus bupivacaine (Marcaine) or ropivacaine (Naropin) • Two separate pain relief techniques are used at one time. • With a "needle-through-needle technique," narcotics are given in the spinal space early in labor. Later, an anesthetic can be dripped continuously via a catheter (thin tube) into the epidural space. No needles, but only a catheter, remain in the mother's back after the initial procedure. • Given as early as 2 cm dilation with narcotics and 6 cm with anesthetic.	• Pain relief throughout labor, with the ability to move (and perhaps walk a bit) in early labor, and without mental effects. • Rest for an exhausted mother.	*Mother:* From the narcotic, itching, nausea and vomiting, retained urine, some weakness in the legs. From the anesthetic, fever, impaired movement in the legs, slowing of labor and the baby's descent, drop in blood pressure, impaired urge and ability to push. *Fetus:* From the anesthetic, heart-rate changes, caused by the mother's fever and low blood pressure. *Baby:* From the anesthetic, fever and diminished reflexes for a few days. Narcotics are absorbed by the baby, but their effects are unknown.	*Mother:* Restriction of food and drink, intravenous fluids, check of muscle strength in legs before the mother tries to walk, additional medications to control itching and nausea (these may make the mother sleepy or interfere with pain relief), bladder catheter, oxytocin to speed labor. *Baby:* Blood, urine, or spinal-fluid cultures to detect infection, antibiotics, and 48 hours in a special-care nursery for observation if the mother had a fever in labor.

244

GENERAL ANESTHESIA

Inhalation gas: nitrous oxide (Entonox), isoflurane (Furan); injected medication: thiopental (Pentothal), ketamine

- Gases are administered by an anesthesiologist to induce total unconsciousness and total muscle inactivity in the mother. (Stronger concentrations of Entonox are used for total anesthesia than for self-administration.)
- Injected medications are transported into a vein to rapidly induce unconsciousness and total muscle inactivity in the mother.
- With either method, the anesthesiologist provides oxygen and mechanically assists with respiration.
- Used before labor when an elective cesarean is planned, or during labor when an emergency cesarean becomes necessary.

- The most rapid, total pain relief and loss of consciousness, for a rapid emergency cesarean.

Mother: Hallucinations, postoperative excitement, amnesia, vomiting and aspiration of stomach contents, respiratory depression, drops in blood pressure and heart rate.
Fetus: Unconsciousness, slowing of movements and heart rate.
Baby: Depression of the central nervous system and respiration, poor muscle tone, low Apgar scores, need for resuscitation.

Mother: Antacid given right before surgery to neutralize stomach contents; intubation (a tube is placed in the windpipe to protect against aspiration of stomach contents); intravenous muscle relaxants; taping of the eyelids to protect the eyes from damage; electrocardiogram; monitoring of the pulse, blood gas levels, and blood pressure; assistance with breathing; electronic fetal monitoring.
Baby: Resuscitation procedures and equipment to assist breathing and alertness.

Continued on next page

Drug Names, and How and Where Given	Desired Effects	Other Possible Effects	Precautions and Procedures for Safe Use
LOCAL ANESTHESIA			
Paracervical Block mepivacaine (Carbocaine), lidocaine (Xylocaine), chloroprocaine (Nesacaine) • Given as an injection into each side of the dilating cervix. • Given after 5 cm and before 9 cm dilation.	• Short-term localized pain relief with no change in consciousness or ability to move freely. • Quick administration that can be done by the mother's doctor; no anesthesiologist is needed. • Alert baby at birth.	*Mother:* Toxic reaction (rare), sudden decrease in blood pressure. *Fetus:* Profound and sudden fetal heart-rate abnormalities. *Baby:* Reduced muscle tone, fussiness, decreased reflexes.	Frequent blood-pressure and blood-oxygenation checks, intravenous fluids, oxygen mask, continuous electronic fetal monitoring, capability to perform rapid cesarean if the baby has an adverse reaction.
Pudendal Block mepivacaine (Carbocaine), lidocaine (Xylocaine), chloroprocaine (Nesacaine) • Given as an injection into pudendal nerve endings on each side of the vaginal canal. • Used during the second stage before application of forceps or vacuum extractor or before an episiotomy.	• Numbing of the birth canal and relaxation of the pelvic floor, enabling a less painful forceps or vacuum extractor delivery or, sometimes, episiotomy.	*Mother:* Toxic reaction (rare), decrease in blood pressure, diminished urge to push, diminished pelvic floor muscle tone, need for forceps or a vacuum extractor (if this need did not exist already). *Fetus:* Sudden drop in heart rate. *Baby:* Temporary reduction in muscle tone, fussiness, decreased reflexes.	Oxytocin, oxygen, episiotomy, availability of forceps or vacuum extractor for delivery.

Perineal Block
mepivacaine (Carbocaine),
lidocaine (Xylocaine),
chloroprocaine (Nesacaine)

- Given as several injections
  into the perineum and vaginal outlet.
- Used during the second
  stage, before an episiotomy,
  or during the third stage to
  repair an episiotomy or tear.

- Numbing of the perineum.
- Less pain during an episiotomy or stitching.

Mother: Pain from injections,
tearing from swelling if injections are given during the second rather than third stage.
Fetus and Baby: Risks unlikely, since the injections are
given just before or after birth.

None

247

Directions for Using the PMPS

Take plenty of time to go over the PMPS. Use it to help her find the approach to pain relief that best suits her, and to discover the kind of help she will need from you to make it work. In the left column the numbers from +10 down to +3 indicate degrees of desire to use pain medication, with +10 being the highest possible (and unrealistic) desire to use them for maximum relief of pain or any other sensations. Zero indicates no opinion. The numbers from −3 to −10 indicate degrees of desire to avoid pain medication, with −10 being an impossible extreme, just as +10 is. Although no one can avoid all sensation in labor, or avoid pain medication in all the possible circumstances that could arise in labor, I put the impossible extremes on the scale to give more meaning to the points in between.

After the mother picks the number that reflects her preferences, then you should both look in the right-hand column for the kind of support and preparation she will need. Can you provide this kind of support? If you have doubts, she can either rethink her preferences to be more in line with the kind of support you can provide, or you can get extra help from a doula or loved one. Is she preparing adequately? Make sure she understands that avoiding pain medication requires more preparation than using it.

PAIN MEDICATIONS PREFERENCE SCALE

Rating	What It Means for the Mother	How the Birth Partner Helps
+ 10	• Desire that she feel nothing; desire for anesthesia before labor begins.	• This is an impossible extreme; if the mother says she is +10, she has no interest in helping herself in labor. Help her accept that it is neither wise nor possible to labor without any feeling. The risks make such a choice highly undesirable. She will have some pain and should focus on dealing with it. • Review the discussion of pain medications with her. • Help her get pain medications as soon as possible.
+ 9	• Fear of pain; lack of confidence that she will be able to cope; dependence on staff to provide total pain relief.	• Follow recommendations for +10. • Suggest she discuss her fears with her caregiver.
+ 7	• Definite desire for anesthesia during labor as soon as the doctor will allow it, or before labor becomes painful.	• Be sure the doctor is aware of her desire for early anesthesia; learn whether having it is possible in your hospital. • Inform staff of her desire when you arrive.
+ 5	• Desire for epidural anesthesia in active labor (at 4 to 5 centimeters dilation). • Willingness to cope until then, perhaps with narcotic medications.	• Encourage her in breathing and relaxation. • Know the comfort measures (page 95). • Suggest medications to her as she approaches active labor.
+ 3	• Desire to use medications—such as a very light epidural or narcotics—to reduce pain rather than to take way all sensation. • Natural childbirth is not a goal.	• Plan to be active as a birth partner to help her keep medication use low. Use comfort measures (page 95). • Help her get medications when she wants them. • Suggest reduced doses of narcotics or a "light" epidural block (to numb the abdomen only).
0	• No opinion or preference. • This attitude is rare among pregnant women, though not among birth partners.	• Become informed. • Discuss medications. • Help her decide what she prefers. • If she has no preference, let the staff manage her pain.

Continued on next page

Rating	What It Means for the Mother	How the Birth Partner Helps
– 3	• Would like to avoid pain medications unless coping becomes difficult, in which case she would feel like a "martyr" if she did not get medications.	• Do not suggest that she take pain medications. • Emphasize coping techniques, but do not try to talk her out of pain medications if she asks for them.
– 5	• Strong preference to avoid pain medications, to avoid side effects on the baby or the labor. • Will accept medications for a long or difficult labor.	• Prepare yourself for a very active role. • If possible, hire a doula to accompany and help the two of you. • When calling the hospital before going in, ask for a nurse who supports natural childbirth. • Learn and practice relaxation techniques, patterned breathing, and massage together in advance. • During labor, do not suggest medications. • If she asks for medications, try other alternatives: Have her checked for progress; ask her to try three to five more contractions without medication; remain firm, confident, and kind; use the Take-Charge Routine (page 134); maintain eye contact and talk her through each contraction.
– 7	• Very strong desire for natural childbirth, for a sense of personal gratification as well as to benefit the baby and the progress of labor. • Will be disappointed if she needs to use medication.	• Follow the recommendations for –5, but with even greater commitment. • Interpret requests for pain medication as expressions of discouragement and a need for more help. • Remind the mother of how much she had wanted an unmedicated birth. • Prearrange for her to use a "last resort" code word if she feels she has had enough and truly wants medication. If she doesn't use the code word, keep encouraging her.

Rating	What It Means for the Mother	How the Birth Partner Helps
– 9	• Desire that you and the staff deny the mother pain medication, even if she requests it.	• Follow the recommendations for –7. • Denying the mother's requests for pain medication would be very difficult if she is in serious pain. You may even be unable to do it. Promise to help all you can, but remind the mother that the final decision is not yours—it is hers. • Explore her reasons for this request.
– 10	• Desire that the mother forego all medications, even for cesarean delivery.	• This is an impossible extreme. Encourage her to learn about complications that require painful interventions. Help her develop a realistic understanding of risks and benefits of pain medications.

WHEN CAN PAIN MEDICATION BE USED?

Medication	First Stage			Second Stage (pushing birth)	Third Stage (placenta)
	Prelabor to 3 cm	*4 to 7 cm*	*8 to 10 cm*		
Morphine (S)	▽————				
Sedatives (S)	▽————				
Tranquilizers (S)	▽	▽	▽————		
Narcotic-like analgesics (S)		▽	▽————		
Narcotic antagonists (S)			▽	▽	▽(to baby)▽
Paracervical block (L)		▽	▽————		
Self-administered inhalation analgesia (S)		▽	▽	▽	▽
Epidural or spinal narcotic analgesia (R)	▽	▽	▽	▽	
Standard epidural anesthesia—with or without narcotics (R)		▽- -			
Segmental ("light and late") epidural anesthesia (R)		▽- -			
Pudendal block (L)				▽	
Perineal block (L)				▽	
Spinal, for cesarean only (R)*	▽- - - - - - - - -		▽	▽- - - - - - - - -	
General anesthesia, for cesarean only (S)*	▽- - - - - - - - -		▽	▽- - - - - - - - -	

*These can be given whenever a cesarean is decided upon.

KEY

———— Time when drug may safely remain in effect.
- - - - - - Time when dosing may be continuous.
▽ Time when drug may be given (some must be discontinued early to allow side effects to diminish before birth).
S systemic medication   R regional anesthesia   L local anesthesia

9

Cesarean Birth, and Vaginal Birth After Cesarean

Sometimes a baby is delivered surgically, through an incision in the mother's abdomen, instead of vaginally. This procedure is a cesarean section, also called cesarean delivery, cesarean birth, C-section, or, simply, a cesarean. Today approximately 23 percent of babies born in the United States and Canada are delivered by cesarean. In fact, cesarean section is the most common surgery performed in U.S. hospitals. The cesarean rate has increased greatly since 1970, when it was 5.5 percent.

The rapid rise in the cesarean rate has undoubtedly improved some outcomes for many mothers and babies. For example, the incidence of forceps-related injuries declined markedly after 1970, when cesareans began replacing many difficult and injurious forceps deliveries. But numerous cesareans are done without medical justification—that is, they do not improve the outcome for either mother or baby. In these cases, a cesarean causes more harm than vaginal birth. Because a cesarean is major surgery, it carries all the same risk—hemorrhage, infection, prolonged healing, adhesions, and others—as other types of major surgery.

Furthermore, prolonged and painful recovery from a cesarean adds challenges (though not insurmountable ones) for the new mother, whose baby needs her night and day. After the surgery, a mother may appreciate that she and the baby are alive and healthy, but at the same time she may feel depressed or disappointed in herself, or upset with her caregivers, especially if she feels the cesarean was avoidable or unnecessary.

Over the past three decades, the medical literature has debated the appropriate use of the cesarean section. The public has joined in, both with organizations formed to halt unnecessary cesareans by teaching about the overuse of the procedure, and with groups that argue for a woman's right to choose whether or not she will avoid labor by having a cesarean. The obstetric profession is divided on the issue; some obstetricians advocate even higher cesarean rates, and others try very hard to perform cesareans only when necessary for the health of mother or baby. Individual doctors' cesarean rates range from 10 to 50 percent of deliveries, with most falling between 14 and 30 percent. Midwives and family physicians generally have lower cesarean rates, with excellent outcomes, than do most obstetricians, even if only the obstetricians' "low-risk" cases (healthy women with healthy pregnancies) are counted. There are also many obstetricians, however, who combine excellent outcomes with low cesarean rates.

The question for health policy makers and consumer groups is this: How high should the cesarean rate be? Some years ago, Healthy People 2000, a government-sponsored panel of U.S. health experts, published specific goals, based on the best scientific evidence, for improving the overall health of Americans by the year 2000. One goal was to reduce the cesarean rate to 15 percent or lower. The panel offered concrete suggestions for doing so. The goal was not achieved, and now Healthy People 2010 has set a goal of 15 percent for first cesareans only by 2010.

The questions for you and the birthing woman are more personal. Can the two of you do anything to avoid a cesarean? Under what circumstances might she still need one, after you have done all you can to lessen the likelihood?

To help you in your role as her birth partner, you need answers to the following questions: What if the need for a cesarean arises during labor? How can you help the mother face it and get through it? What can you do to ensure that she has as good an experience as possible, despite this unexpected turn of events? How might you feel during this mysterious, highly technological procedure involving the woman and baby you care for so deeply? This chapter will give you some answers to these questions.

Avoiding a Cesarean. Many women, if they have a choice, seek caregivers with low cesarean rates for women who are at low risk of complications, and choose birth settings in which cesarean rates are low. Additionally, learning techniques to relieve pain and enhance labor progress, participating in decision making (see the "Key Questions" on page 171), and having a doula are ways to improve the chances of a vaginal birth.

Know the Reasons for Cesarean Birth

Both you and the mother should understand the reasons for the cesarean before it is done and agree that it is the right thing to do. If she finds out in advance that she or the baby has a medical problem that requires a cesarean delivery or makes it highly likely, she can learn all about the surgery and adjust emotionally beforehand. If the need for the cesarean arises in labor, she will have to do much of the adjusting afterwards. Either way, she should have plenty of opportunity to talk about the experience with you, the doctor, and the nurses.

See chapters 6 and 7 for information about problems that sometimes arise in labor and how they are detected and treated; a cesarean becomes the solution if other treatments are unsuccessful.

Following are the most likely reasons for a cesarean. Whereas cesareans are not always necessary in these circumstances, they are always considered and very often done.

1. *Emergencies.* These include the following:
• Prolapsed cord (page 213).
• Serious hemorrhage (excessive bleeding) in the mother (page 208).

In these situations there is no time for questions. Rapid action is essential.

2. *Arrested labor.* This is the most common reason for a woman's first cesarean. A failure to progress in labor may be caused by the following:

- Abnormal position or presentation of the baby.
- Uterine inertia.
- A poor fit between the baby's head and the mother's pelvis (see page 211).
- A combination of these.

According to many experts, far too many cesareans are performed because of arrested labor (see "Problems with Labor Progress," page 209).

3. *Problems with the fetus.* These include the following:

- Fetal distress. Many experts believe this is another reason for which cesareans are too often performed (see "Fetal Distress," page 216).
- Breech presentation (when the baby's buttocks or feet will be born first), combined with large size and other factors. Vaginal breech births are still done in selected cases when the doctor has been trained in the techniques. (See "A Breech Baby," page 160.)
- Prematurity, postmaturity (when the baby is overdue), or other conditions that might make vaginal birth too stressful to the fetus. Through fetal movement counting, by which the mother keeps track of how much the fetus moves (page 23), nonstress testing (page 181), and ultrasound (the use of soundwaves to obtain pictures of the insides of the fetus), the caregiver predicts whether the fetus can tolerate labor.

4. *Problems with the mother.* These include the following:

- Serious illness (such as heart disease, diabetes, or preeclampsia) or injury. Sometimes, in these cases, a cesarean section is planned in advance. Otherwise a "trial of labor" is allowed. The mother is watched carefully and, if all goes well, she gives birth vaginally. If the problem worsens, she has a cesarean.
- A genital herpes sore (see page 205).
- A previous cesarean delivery. This is the primary reason for the

overall high cesarean rate in the United States and Canada. Most women who have had a cesarean before will have another, even though few truly need one. This trend contradicts numerous research findings and the government panels, all of which have stated that few pregnant women who have had cesareans should plan for repeat cesareans. Most of these mothers and their babies would benefit from labor, and most of these women could safely give birth vaginally. (See "A Previous Disappointing Birth Experience," page 163, and "Vaginal Birth After Cesarean," page 265.)

Once the decision to perform a cesarean is made, concentrate on helping the mother and greeting the baby as lovingly and gently as you can.

Know What to Expect During Cesarean Birth

You may be surprised by how quickly the staff moves once the decision is made to do a cesarean, and by the number of people involved: There is the doctor who will do the surgery; an assisting doctor or midwife; a "scrub nurse," who gives instruments to the doctor; a "floating nurse," who prepares the room and looks after the surgical team; an anesthesiologist; a nursery nurse or two to look after the baby; and possibly a pediatrician or neonatologist, if problems with the baby are anticipated. They all work together as an efficient, businesslike team.

You may feel frightened and worried for the mother or baby. You may feel relieved to know that the end is in sight, especially after a long, difficult labor. You may be impressed and reassured by the teamwork and competence of the staff. You may feel left out or even shocked by their apparently casual attitude. They may talk and even joke among themselves, paying little attention to you and the mother, as if you are not there. You may feel overwhelmed by the sounds, smells, and sights of the surgery. You may be confused over your role. Should you ask questions, and try to make sure that the mother's wishes are being followed, or should you stay out of the way and let them proceed in their customary manner? Just a few minutes before, your role was essential to the mother's ability to handle her contractions; now you feel much less important. Be assured that you are still most important to the mother, but in a different way. The following descriptions of the surgery and of your role will help you to help the mother.

Preparations for Surgery

Preparations for cesarean delivery include the following steps:

- The mother signs a consent form.
- A nurse starts intravenous (IV) fluids in the mother's arm, which is placed on a board that extends out to the side. The nurse checks the mother's blood pressure frequently.
- The mother may be given a sedative. She can refuse it if she wants to remain aware during the surgery and immediately after birth.
- An anesthesiologist, nurse-anesthetist, or obstetrician gives the anesthetic (spinal, epidural, or general; see chapter 8). The choice of anesthesia depends on the mother's situation, the training and qualifications of the staff, and the facilities. General anesthesia, being fastest, is chosen if the cesarean must be done immediately, but regional anesthesia is safer under most circumstances. Regulating bodies require that hospitals be able to provide general anesthesia, but not necessarily regional anesthesia, around the clock.
- The mother will probably receive oxygen, administered with a face mask or nasal prongs (tubes that blow oxygen into the nose).
- Electrocardiogram (EKG) leads are placed on her chest. These keep track of the mother's heart rate throughout the surgery.
- The mother's body is draped so that only her abdomen can be seen. The end of the drape is raised to form a screen between her head and her abdomen. Even if she is conscious, she cannot see the surgery.
- Most hospitals now welcome the mother's birth partner (or partners) in the operating room for a cesarean. You sit on a stool at her head. The anesthesiologist remains at her head also.
- Some birth partners want to watch and even photograph the

surgery. Discuss this option with the mother and her caregiver, if it interests you. If you remain sitting on the stool, you will see nothing. You will have to stand up and look over the drape in order to see the surgery.

- The mother's abdomen is scrubbed and shaved. Some pubic hair is usually removed.
- A catheter is placed in her bladder to keep it empty.

Surgery Begins

This is how a cesarean delivery starts:

- Once the anesthetic takes effect, the doctor makes the incisions with a scalpel.
- The skin incision is usually low and horizontal, or *transverse* (this is called a "bikini incision"), but occasionally is vertical and in the midabdomen.
- The muscles of the abdomen are not cut; they are separated from each other and spread apart. The muscles therefore heal very well.
- The uterine incision is usually horizontal (transverse) in the lower segment of the uterus, but it can be made higher if speed is essential or if the higher opening is needed to get the baby out (for example, in the case of twins or an unusual presentation).
- The amniotic fluid is suctioned from the uterus. You will hear the sucking sound.
- To prevent excessive bleeding, the cut blood vessels are cauterized. You may hear the high-pitched tone of the cautery device or notice a slight odor as it burns the ends of the blood vessels to close them. The mother cannot feel this.
- If at any time during the procedure the mother indicates that she is feeling pain, make sure the doctor knows it and stops working until more anesthetic can be given. This does not happen often, but sometimes the anesthesia is spotty and the mother is not numb where she needs to be.

The Baby Is Born

This is how the baby is delivered:

- The baby is usually delivered within 15 minutes after the surgery has begun. The doctor places one hand in the uterus;

KNOW WHAT TO EXPECT DURING CESAREAN BIRTH

the assisting doctor pushes on the mother's abdomen to move the baby to the incision. The first doctor removes the baby. The mother may feel pressure and tugging, but should not feel pain. Help her to use relaxation and patterned breathing (page 102), and ask the doctor or anesthesiologist if she can have more anesthetic.

• The doctor or nurse suctions the baby's airways, and clamps and cuts the cord. You may want to ask the doctor to lower the drape so the mother can see the baby, or the baby may be briefly held up for you both to admire. Then he is taken to an infant-care area in the corner of the delivery room, or in an adjacent room, for evaluation and any necessary treatment. By this time he is probably crying lustily. You may wish to go over and take a look at the baby.

• The oxygen apparatus is removed from the mother's face.

You will probably be allowed to get close to the baby, to see him, talk to him, and possibly stroke him or hold his hand. The thought of talking to the baby many seem strange at first, but you may be able to soothe the baby as no one else can (except his mother, but she cannot be with him). If you are the baby's father or the mother's lover, the baby knows your voice and will respond when he hears it. Think of this birth from the baby's point of view—an abrupt tug out of his mother's warm and familiar womb to a bright, cold, noisy place. He is handled competently, but perfunctorily, and only hears strangers' voices. Then you come close and say, "Hi, Baby! I'm so glad to see you. Everything is all right and I'm here to take care of you." You stroke his arm and put your finger into the palm of his hand. He stares into your eyes and clings to your finger. At last, a familiar voice and loving touch for the baby! You will never forget this moment.

The Placenta Is Removed and the Uterus Is Inspected

While you are greeting the baby, the doctor completes the delivery:

• The doctor reaches into the uterus, separates the placenta from the wall of the uterus, and removes it.

- Some doctors then lift the uterus out of the abdomen to check it thoroughly. The mother may feel this as uncomfortable pressure. She may feel nauseated and vomit, turning her head to the side and using the basin that you or the anesthesiologist holds for her. Because the benefit of removing the uterus is questionable, and because it causes the mother discomfort, many physicians have stopped doing it.

The Repair Begins

The repair phase takes about 30 to 45 minutes. These procedures are involved:

- The uterus and other internal layers are sutured with absorbable suture thread.
- The skin is closed with stitches or stainless steel clips. You may hear the clicking of the stapler as the clips are placed.
- A bandage is applied over the incision.
- Since the mother may be very shaky, trembling all over, or nauseated, she might be given a relaxing, sleep-inducing medication via her IV line—without either of you knowing about it. If it is important to her to be awake after the birth so she can experience the first hours with her baby, you should ask ahead of time, and again just after the birth, that these medications not be given without first checking with her. The nausea and trembling usually subside within a half hour.

  If the nausea and trembling are extreme, she can always change her mind and ask for some medication. It takes effect within 2 minutes.

  There is one medication, Versed, that she should be warned about. Along with being an effective sedative, it is also a potent amnesiac. It wipes out all memory of the birth and events for hours afterwards. The mother will not remember having the baby, nor will she remember her first impressions or the first feeding. There are other sedatives that do not do this. The absence of memory of the momentous event might haunt her and cause much regret.
- The mother is cleaned up and taken to the recovery area. Most hospitals have a multi-bed recovery room; others simply return a woman to her labor room after a cesarean.

KNOW WHAT TO EXPECT DURING CESAREAN BIRTH

The Recovery Period

This is what you can expect during the recovery period:

- The mother remains in recovery for a few hours, until it is clear that she is recovering well and that the anesthetic is wearing off as expected. The baby may remain with the mother or go to the nursery for observation or treatment.
- The nurse frequently checks the mother's pulse, temperature, blood pressure, uterine tone, and state of anesthesia.
- The mother and baby may be separated. In this case, where should you be? If you stay with the mother, you can comfort her and ease your worries about her. But both of you may wonder how the baby is doing or worry that he may be crying. If you go with the baby, then you can soothe him and perhaps take some photos, and you will be able later to tell the mother what happened when she could not be with him. But then you may worry about how the mother is doing. This is a difficult choice. If a family member or doula can stay with one, then you can be with the other, and have some peace of mind.
- The mother can breastfeed the baby now. She will need the nurses to help her to position the baby and get started. It is a good idea for her to begin breastfeeding before the anesthesia wears off, since it will be a little easier for her to get started when she is not in pain. She may need your help in holding the baby up to the breast.
- If she is asleep or groggy from the medication for nausea and trembling, it will be hard for her to nurse. This is why some women refuse medication for nausea and trembling, preferring to put up with it for a half-hour to an hour: They do not want to miss the first few hours with the baby.
- If the mother is unable to nurse or hold the baby, you take him. Hold the baby close and talk to him.
- The nurse checks the baby's breathing, skin color, temperature, and heart rate frequently.
- Once the anesthesia wears off and the mother's condition is stable, she is taken to her postpartum room, where she will stay until she goes home. See chapter 10 for information about the first few days after birth.

Your Role During Cesarean Birth

Few women prefer to give birth by cesarean. For most, a cesarean is unexpected and disappointing, even when they know the surgery has made possible the birth of a healthy baby. Some get over these feelings quickly; others do not. A woman often needs time afterward to adjust emotionally, to talk about and even grieve over the experience, especially if she had a strong desire to give birth vaginally. It is sometimes surprising to loved ones, nurses, and caregivers how deeply disappointed some mothers are. The mother may need much patience and understanding from you to help her come to terms with her baby's cesarean birth.

The mother is less likely to grieve for a long time if she has been able to participate thoroughly in her labor and in the decision to have a cesarean. Prolonged anger, depression, or guilt may come if the mother is caught by surprise and can do nothing to help herself or make decisions. How you respond to the mother, both during and after the cesarean, also makes a big difference in how well she adjusts. Here are guidelines:

- Your perceptions of what has happened will be very important to the mother as she puts the pieces together. You can help her come to terms with the experience later if, during the surgery, you stay with her, ask questions, hold her hand, and try to keep her posted on what is happening. You may want to take some pictures; many women, especially if they were unaware during the surgery, treasure photographs of it later. They help to fill her in on the parts she missed. Even if she has no interest in photos of the surgery, early pictures of her baby will probably mean a great deal to her.

- The mother, if aware, will probably feel some discomfort during the surgery. If she feels pain as well as pressure or tugging, ask that she be given more anesthetic. You should help her continue her relaxation and patterned breathing to handle the sensations of pressure and tugging.

- After birth, do as much as you can with the baby. If possible, hold the baby where the mother can see, touch, or kiss him. Help her breastfeed in recovery. If the baby has to go to the nursery for special care, you may want to go along so that you can see for yourself what is being done and fill in these gaps for the mother later. Or, the mother may want you to stay with her.

- It may take the mother longer to recover emotionally than it takes her to recover physically. It will also surely take her longer than it takes you. Be patient. Give her time, and help her to understand what has happened.
- Physical recovery takes a matter of weeks or months. Pain, weakness, and fatigue are great at first, but diminish steadily for the first week or two. Then, it may take months for the last step—from functioning fairly well to returning to how she was before she became pregnant.
- Women vary in how long it takes them to integrate and accept the cesarean birth experience. For some, a cesarean will be a positive experience; for others it will not be. If the mother is disappointed, accept her feelings as valid and normal. Too often a woman's loved ones try to distract her from thinking about the birth by pointing out that "all that matters" is that she has a healthy baby. But that is not all that matters. Her feelings also matter, and her loved ones' patience, acceptance, and concern for these feelings will help her work through them.
- If the mother's birth experience was particularly negative, she may benefit from professional counseling or therapy. Call her caregiver or childbirth educator for referrals. See "Unhappiness After Childbirth," page 295.
- See chapter 7 for more suggestions about the birth partner's role when problems arise during labor.

Despite her possible disappointment with the birth experience, the mother will rejoice in her baby. A cesarean birth is, after all, a birth, and all the emotions that come with birth also come with cesarean birth. The mother's ability to love, feed, enjoy, and care for her baby are not altered by the fact that the baby was born by cesarean. You will enjoy this child together.

Vaginal Birth After Cesarean (VBAC)

With modern surgical techniques, the uterine incision made during a cesarean usually heals well afterwards, and there is a good possibility of a vaginal birth in the future. Sixty to 80 percent of women who attempt a VBAC have one.

Since VBAC is usually safer than a repeat cesarean, and recovery is easier and faster, it is important to begin immediately after the cesarean to create a positive outlook for a future vaginal birth. Before the woman goes home from the hospital, she should be sure to ask the doctor if she has a good chance of a vaginal birth with her next baby. The sooner she hears from "the expert" that she is a good candidate for a VBAC, the better for her state of mind. Most women do not think about future births until they are pregnant again. But those who have carried a positive message in their minds about a possible vaginal birth in the future feel much less anxiety and self-doubt when they become pregnant again. Those who have carried only the message that their bodies did not work have a much harder time regaining confidence in a subsequent pregnancy.

Of course, a small percentage of women have a medical or physical condition or the kind of uterine incision that necessitates another cesarean. It helps for them to know this as well.

Once a woman becomes pregnant after having had a cesarean, she may feel less confident about giving birth than she did when pregnant the first time. She may feel that she was naïve before, and is now realistic enough to recognize that she might have another cesarean this time. Her preparation for a vaginal birth should include exploring emotions involving the cesarean and the upcoming birth, and also seeking out resources that will give her the best chance of a safe and satisfying experience. Once the mother has prepared as well as she can to optimize her chances for a VBAC, she will know that she will give birth vaginally unless a cesarean is truly appropriate.

As the birth partner in such a situation, you may have mixed feelings about trying for a vaginal birth, especially if the mother's first labor was distressing for you. It will help to prepare yourself, so that you can fully support the mother's efforts.

Improving Her Chances for a Vaginal Birth

Obstetricians vary widely in their support of VBACs, and their attitudes are reflected in their repeat cesarean rates. An unsupportive doctor or midwife is likely to warn the woman against getting her hopes up, or to emphasize potential complications, instead of encouraging her. Such a negative attitude may undermine her confidence and lead her, in the words of one woman, "down the garden path to another cesarean."

It is wise for the mother to learn which local hospitals maintain low cesarean rates, and to interview some doctors and midwives who work there. She should check her health plan to find out which caregivers are covered by her insurance. She might also ask a childbirth educator (preferably one who is self-employed, or one who is employed by the hospital she is considering) for advice on which caregivers interview or consult.

If you attend these interviews, you can give her confidence to ask and discuss such questions as: Do you support VBACs? What percentage of your clients who have had cesareans plan to have VBACs? What percentage succeed? Can you recommend ways I can improve my chances for a VBAC? Do your associates share your opinions about VBACs?

After comparing the attitudes of the various caregivers, she can choose one who seems most supportive.

It certainly helps if she is surrounded by people who respect her desire for a VBAC and assume that she can and will do it. Her family and friends, her professional caregivers, and you most of all should have confidence in her. A doula can supply a lot of practical advice and encouragement to you, the mother, and other helpers.

Knowledge of some of the controversies regarding VBAC, of what to expect, and of ways to deal with some of the challenges inherent to VBAC labors will arm both of you with self-confidence and helpful coping strategies. Childbirth classes are valuable preparation. A good refresher class should cover the unique challenges that come with VBACs. There are also valuable books on the subject of vaginal birth after cesarean, and the Internet contains websites and news groups centering on VBAC. Lastly, if the woman suffered emotional or physical trauma in her previous birth experience, counseling with a perinatal social worker, a trauma therapist, a seasoned childbirth educator, or a sensitive midwife or doctor may help her develop strategies to prevent troubling thoughts and feelings from undermining her self-confidence (see "Recommended Resources").

Fears About VBAC

Most VBAC labors proceed normally, even though they carry a small extra risk due to the fact that the uterus bears a scar from the cesarean. The greatest fear about a VBAC is the risk of scar separation, sometimes referred to as uterine rupture. The risk of scar separation ranges between 0.2 and 1.5 percent, and may be somewhat higher in women who have had more than one cesarean. With careful monitoring of the fetal heart rate and observation of the mother, however, uterine rupture usually can be detected in time for a cesarean to be performed and the separation mended. Though worrisome when they occur, most scar separations end well, with a healthy mother and baby, because of immediate and appropriate action.

A uterine scar sometimes thins during labor without separating, but when this happens, the uterus heals itself as it returns to its nonpregnant state.

If the mother wants a VBAC, help her take some important steps in preparation:

- Explore any strong emotions associated with the first cesarean. Was it necessary? Was it traumatic? Was she well cared for?
- Explore any fears about the next labor—a fear of pain or exhaustion, or a fear that something could go wrong (the scar could separate, she could have another cesarean, or she could encounter a lack of support from her caregiver, the nurses, or even from you).
- Explore her feelings about her caregiver and the hospital where she gave birth. Does she want to go back to them? Were they a part of the problem? Can she find a caregiver whom she trusts?
- Explore how much she wants a VBAC. Is she willing to prepare herself not only with these steps, but also by learning self-help measures for comfort and aiding labor progress? Is she willing to use medications and other interventions very

judiciously? Will she surround herself with truly supportive friends and relatives?

Special Challenges During a VBAC

Beyond the usual emotional challenges that come with most labors (see chapter 3), a woman having a VBAC may have to deal with other challenges.

As she enters labor, she may feel extra anxiety; this may be her "moment of truth," when her courage and conviction will be put to the test. This normal reaction may trouble both of you and fill her with self-doubt, unless she has anticipated such feelings and made a plan with you for dealing with them (for example, by talking about them with you; having you remind her that early labor jitters are expected, and that her job is to carry on in spite of them; and by guarding against overreacting to the contractions out of fear).

Flashbacks to her previous labor could sap her confidence. You can prevent this by helping her separate last time from this time. For example, she may hope her membranes will not rupture before labor as they did the first time. If they do, she might interpret the rupture as a bad omen. By talking about this, you can help her recognize that early rupture is not predictive of a cesarean. You may prevent her fear from becoming a self-fulfilling prophesy.

If you, as her birth partner, have flashbacks to the previous labor, it is best that you talk to someone else about them. Do not increase her anxiety with your own. If you have a doula, you might talk with her; if not, you might talk to the nurse, out of earshot of the laboring woman. If the doula or nurse knows you are troubled, she can reassure you in nonverbal ways.

The point in labor (in centimeters of dilation or number of hours) when the mother had her cesarean may represent a big emotional hurdle. Until she gets past it, she may have trouble seeing this labor as different from the last. If so, passing the hurdle will bring new optimism. Of course, this does not apply to the woman who had a planned cesarean without labor, or the woman who had a cesarean after pushing for three hours!

Reluctance to Try for a VBAC

For a woman who has had a long exhausting labor that ended in a cesarean, the thought of attempting a VBAC may raise all kinds of fear. "I can't put myself through all that again," she may say. "I'd rather just plan a cesarean." After a traumatic or disappointing first labor, she may be very reluctant to try again, even though she may dread the thought of having to recover from major surgery while taking care of an infant and a toddler.

In such a situation, you might suggest that she think about circumstances under which she would be willing to labor—for example, if she doesn't have to push again for three hours, or if she doesn't have to keep going after her labor stalls for more than two hours. If she concludes that she would prefer to try for a VBAC as long as she does not have to go through an ordeal like the first birth, then she might discuss the idea with her caregiver, and prepare a birth plan for a VBAC that reflects the limits that she and her caregiver set. Knowing that this labor will not be allowed to happen as the first one did, she then can put her mind at rest and focus on a positive birth experience over which she has some control.

Part Four
AFTER THE BIRTH

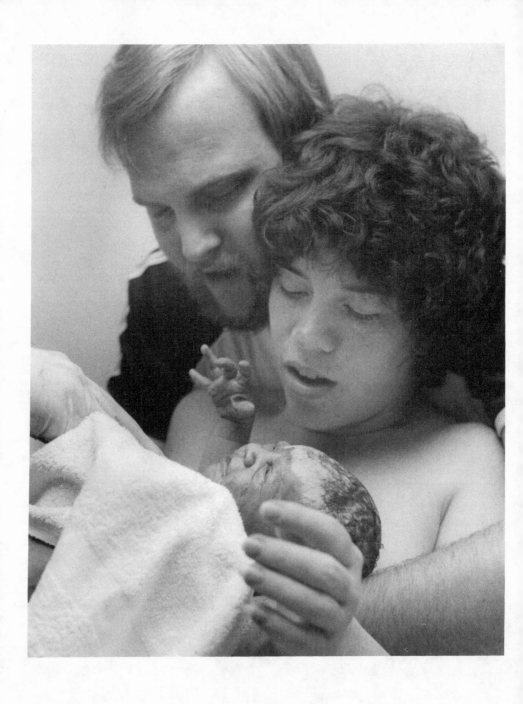

ONCE THE BABY AND THE PLACENTA ARE BORN, the pace seems to slow down. Everyone relaxes. The caregiver and the staff seem preoccupied with finishing the medical tasks and with cleaning up. You, the mother, and the baby are almost in your own world, engrossed with the appearance, the touch, the smell of one another. The baby's every gurgle, every grimace, every squirming stretch brings fascinated exclamations and surprised looks from both of you. Some babies are quiet, calm, and alert, drinking in all the new sights and sounds, the most captivating being your faces and your voices. Other babies fuss and cry a lot at first as they discover themselves in strange new surroundings. They seem to need soothing and reassurance right away.

If you are the father of the baby or the mother's life partner, this is the beginning of a "honeymoon" for the three of you. What happens is much like a honeymoon between lovers: withdrawal from the everyday events of the world, intense preoccupation and fascination with each other, profound feelings of love, lack of sleep, and deep contentment.

If your involvement with the mother is as a labor-support person only, your contact with her may not extend beyond the birth and a few hours afterward. Make sure the mother has someone else with her during this adjustment period, because she still needs help. You might want to pass this book along to the "at home" support person(s). Chapters 10 and 11, which follow, have some helpful information about the postpartum period and breastfeeding.

10

The First Few Days Postpartum

*D*uring the first few days after the birth, there is much going on physically, medically, and emotionally with both the mother and the baby. This chapter explains what to expect in the first few hours and days—what the caregiver does, what happens with the mother and baby, and your role in all this. Your primary role, of course, is to stay with the mother and give her as much emotional support and practical help as possible.

The First Few Hours

Immediately after the birth, the baby is quickly checked and (assuming all is well) dried and placed naked against the mother's skin. Both are covered with warm blankets. This skin-to-skin contact is really the best way to keep the baby warm—better than wrapping the baby warmly. The baby may be crying or may be accustoming herself quietly to her new surroundings. You and the mother will probably be focused completely on the baby, except when reality reenters in the form of the caregiver's or nurse's

275

necessary intrusions. Their agenda is a little different from yours: Their main concern is the physical well-being of the mother and the baby. So, while the two of you are engrossed in the baby, they are dealing with the following immediate clinical concerns.

The Mother's Vagina and Perineum

After a vaginal birth the caregiver carefully inspects the mother's vagina and perineum to determine whether stitches are necessary. This examination is often quite painful if the mother has had no anesthesia. An episiotomy (page 195) or a sizeable tear will require stitches. The caregiver gives the mother a local anesthetic if she needs stitches and if she is not already anesthetized. The stitches are gradually absorbed as the incision heals; they do not have to be removed.

After a Cesarean

After a cesarean birth (described in chapter 9), the mother leaves the operating room and spends a few hours in the recovery room or in her labor room while the anesthetic wears off. She may be very sleepy, depending on the drugs she has been given. There will be a nurse close by all the time. You can remain with the mother, and unless the baby has a problem that requires care in the nursery, he can probably stay, too.

The Mother's Uterus

The mother's uterus is checked frequently by the nurse to be sure it is contracting tightly. If it is soft and relaxed, it will bleed too much. There are three ways to make it contract:

- *Nipple stimulation.* When the baby suckles, the hormone oxytocin is released, which makes the uterus contract. If the baby is not ready to suckle, you or the mother can stroke or roll the mother's nipples, which has almost the same effect.
- *Fundal massage.* The nurse or the midwife does this, but the mother can learn to do it, too. This massage involves firmly kneading the low abdomen until the uterus contracts to the size and consistency of a large grapefruit. This is painful for the mother, which is one reason she should learn to do it her-

self: She can do it less vigorously and get the same results.

• *Injection or intravenous administration of Pitocin or Methergine.* This is the most reliable way to contract the uterus; it may be used along with the methods described above, although it is not needed in most cases.

The Mother's and Baby's Vital Signs

The caregiver frequently checks the vital signs (pulse, respiration, temperature, and blood pressure) of the mother and the baby, as well as performing other routine assessments. Of course, if the mother or the baby had medical problems during the pregnancy or labor, the nurse or caregiver watches even more closely. The nurse or midwife will also check the mother's lochia (see page 287).

Common Procedures in Newborn Care

In the first few minutes or hours after birth, the newborn is examined and a number of procedures are done. Many of these are routine; others are optional; some are required by law to detect or prevent certain serious conditions. Because the mother may be exhausted or preoccupied with the things that are still happening to her, it will be up to you to keep track of what is being done to the baby, remind the staff of the mother's preferences regarding newborn care, and help the mother make decisions, if necessary.

Suctioning the Baby's Nose and Mouth. There are two ways to suck mucus, amniotic fluid, or blood from the baby's airway:

1. The tip of a rubber bulb syringe is inserted into the baby's nostrils and mouth, as soon as the head is out or when the baby is born. Most caregivers do this to all newborns in their practice because it is quick and simple and seems to have few harmful side effects. Some, however, wait to see if the baby needs it.

2. Sometimes, deeper suctioning is done with a long tube that is passed through a nostril and down the baby's trachea (windpipe).

Purposes of Suctioning. Suctioning is done to clear the airway of secretions, especially if the baby is unable to cough or sneeze to remove them, or to assist the baby who is not breathing.

Deeper suctioning may be done if the baby has had a meconium bowel movement while still in the uterus, to keep the baby from breathing the meconium into the lungs. Because the meconium may be in the airway, the caregiver tries to suction it out before the baby's first breath, and again as soon as possible after the birth. Occasionally, however, a baby breathes in meconium before the head is out.

Disadvantages of Suctioning. These are (1) brief discomfort and stress for the baby, who may flinch or struggle when it is done; and (2) possible abrasions of mucous membranes in the baby's nose and throat if the tip scrapes them.

Alternatives to Consider. You and the mother can ask the caregiver to withhold suctioning unless the baby is unable to rid his airway of secretions. If suctioning is necessary, the caregiver can use the syringe gently.

Eye Medication. An antibiotic (usually erythromycin ointment) is placed in the baby's eyes within the first hour after birth.

Purposes of Eye Medication. The antibiotic prevents serious eye infection or even blindness due to bacteria that cause gonorrhea or chlamydia, two common sexually transmitted diseases. These bacteria are sometimes present in the vagina and can be transmitted to the baby during birth.

Eye medication is medically indicated if the mother tests positive for chlamydia or gonorrhea or if either parent may have been exposed to the diseases (by having sex with someone else). Because lab tests can miss these infections, medication is required by all states and provinces unless the parent refuses it and the nurse (or other person required to give it) agrees to withhold it from the baby.

Disadvantages of Eye Medication. The medicine temporarily blurs the baby's vision.

Alternatives to Eye Medication. Refusal may be risky, because the organisms, especially chlamydia, are very prevalent and are not always tested for during pregnancy. Because chlamydia and gonorrhea organisms do not always cause symptoms in adults, they sometimes go untreated. Unfortunately, the newborn can be seriously infected by these organisms. Your nurse or caregiver may feel very uncomfortable if you refuse, since many states hold the caregiver responsible if eye treatment is not given and the baby develops one of these infections.

Another alternative is to ask the nurse or midwife to postpone putting the ointment in the baby's eyes until an hour after birth, so the baby will be able to see your faces clearly in the meantime.

Vitamin K. Required in most U.S. states and Canadian provinces, vitamin K is given as an injection or oral dose within an hour after birth. This vitamin is essential in the clotting of blood. Newborns are relatively slow in clotting their blood for the first week or so, although once they start eating and digesting food they begin making their own vitamin K. Until then, they are at risk for excessive bleeding (called *hemorrhagic disease of the newborn*). Giving them vitamin K to tide them over reduces the risk of bleeding problems.

Most hospitals and doctors give vitamin K only by injection, but giving it by mouth has been approved by the American Academy of Pediatrics and the Canadian Paediatric Society. The injection is given once, in the thigh. Oral vitamin K is given after birth, at one to two weeks of age, and again at four weeks of age.

Purposes of Giving Vitamin K. The vitamin is given

- Whenever internal bleeding is more likely than usual, as in a difficult forceps birth.
- When the baby is premature.
- When circumcision or other surgery is planned before the baby is a week old.
- Routinely in the United States and Canada, because it is quick, easy, and inexpensive to give, and very effective in preventing hemorrhagic disease.

Disadvantages of Giving Vitamin K. These are

- The injection is briefly painful.

- Administered orally, vitamin K does not taste good, and it has to be given carefully to be sure that the baby swallows it.
- Large doses of vitamin K have been associated with newborn jaundice (see page 222).

Alternatives to Giving Vitamin K. You and the mother may ask the hospital, your baby's doctor, or your midwife for the less traumatic oral administration of vitamin K. Refusing vitamin K altogether is a risky option, because it is not possible to predict which babies will or will not develop hemorrhagic disease.

Blood Tests. Blood samples are obtained in two ways:

1. A few drops of the baby's blood are drawn from the heel or a vein to check for

- The level of bilirubin, a yellowish blood pigment that at high levels causes jaundice.
- Blood sugar (glucose) levels.
- Rare disorders that cause mental retardation if left untreated, such as PKU (phenylketonuria) and congenital hypothyroidism. Low levels of particular substances in the blood indicate these disorders.
- Infection, if the mother had a fever in labor or if the baby has one now.

2. Blood from the baby's umbilical cord may also be collected at birth, for

- Blood typing.
- Rh determination.
- Storage or donation to a blood bank (see page 87).

Purposes of Blood Tests. The general purpose of testing the newborn's blood is to detect potentially serious problems early enough to treat them and prevent dangerous effects on the baby.

The PKU test is required for all babies in North America. If the first test indicates PKU, a second test is done, and, if appropriate, a special diet is prescribed.

Other tests may be performed if the baby is at risk for any of certain disorders, as determined by family history and the course of the pregnancy or the postpartum period.

Disadvantages of Blood Tests. The heel stick or blood draw is painful to the baby, and some of the tests (such as those for bilirubin and blood glucose) may have to be repeated many times.

Also, results of blood tests are sometimes confusing and can lead to overtreatment. Experts sometimes disagree on the interpretation of the results and the appropriate course of action. For example, the question of when bilirubin and blood glucose levels are dangerous is the subject of controversy. Ask the "Key Questions" (see page 171) to learn enough to make a good decision about any recommended tests.

Alternatives to Consider. You and the mother can ask the caregiver about less painful ways to gain the information provided by blood tests. For example, you can observe the baby's skin and the whites of his eyes, and do a blood test for jaundice only if they appear yellow. Weigh the risks and benefits of the recommended test and the problem it is designed to detect, and then make informed choices.

If a blood test shows a problem requiring treatment, such as jaundice or low blood sugar (*hypoglycemia*), you can seek a second opinion. If the second caregiver interprets the test results in the same way as the first, you may be reassured that treatment is necessary. If the two opinions disagree, you and the mother can follow the one that makes the most sense to you.

Warming Unit. A warming unit is a special bed with a heater above it. A baby who is placed in a warming unit has a small thermostat taped to her abdomen; the thermostat automatically turns up the heat if the baby gets chilled. Small or premature babies get chilled more easily than average-sized or full-term babies.

Purposes of the Warming Unit. The unit is used to prevent a temperature drop and its harmful aftereffects (sluggishness, increased blood sugar, lung problems, and others), or to warm a baby who has become chilled.

Disadvantages of the Warming Unit. The baby is separated from her parents. Also, warming units are not risk-free; they cause the baby to lose fluids. This fluid loss must be monitored carefully, and the fluids replaced.

Alternatives to Consider. To prevent chills, dry the baby right after the birth and don't leave her exposed to the air. Keep her warm by placing her skin-to-skin against her mother and covering her with a hat and blanket, or by wrapping her snugly in a warm blanket.

Cleanup

The mother's bed is changed; the caregiver or the nurse helps the mother wash up and put on a clean gown. The mother should make sure the gown opens in the front for convenience in breastfeeding. The mother wears a sanitary napkin to catch the bloody vaginal discharge, or lochia (see page 287), which will be present for several days or weeks. The baby is wiped clean, dressed, and diapered. The baby should wear a hat (which you or the hospital supplies). A hat helps keep the baby warm all over; when his head is uncovered, heat is lost from his entire body.

During all this cleanup activity, the mother should hold the baby close to her breast so that he can nurse as soon as he is ready. The nurse or the midwife can be a great help in getting the baby to "latch on" to the breast correctly. Ask for help if the baby is having difficulty or if the mother is unsure of what to do. See chapter 11 for more on breastfeeding.

When the immediate postpartum care is over, the mother, the baby, and the birth partner are often left alone for a while in peace and quiet. Dim the lights to encourage the baby to open his eyes; enjoy these quiet moments together. You and the mother both will soon be ready for a meal. If the mother had a cesarean delivery, it might be some time before she is offered anything more than clear liquids. She may continue receiving IV fluids for up to a day after the cesarean.

The Next Few Days for the Baby

In the first hours after birth, the mother and baby are checked over and cleaned up. Once both mother and baby are settled, the three of you can relax together, cooing, cuddling, exploring, and nursing—or simply sleeping. There is usually no reason for mothers and babies to be separated after birth, although for a long time it was (and still is in some places) a hospital custom to separate them. If the mother or baby is not well, the baby may go to the nursery or the mother may be unable to hold her.

You are the perfect person to hold the baby if the mother cannot (and even if she can), or to remain with the baby in the nursery, as long as both you and the mother wish for you to do so.

Physical Exam and Assessment

A doctor or a midwife will give the baby a thorough physical exam, checking her entire body and all her systems. It is interesting to watch the exam, which can teach you a great deal about the baby. Over the next few days you, the mother, or the staff will make certain observations of the baby: the number and quality of bowel movements, frequency of urination, frequency and length of time in feeding, respiration, temperature, pulse, and so forth. The caregiver will teach you more about these observations if they are to be your responsibility.

Bowel Movements

The baby will have a bowel movement within a few hours after birth. This bowel movement is called meconium, and it is different from later bowel movements. It is black and sticky and hard to clean. If you think of it, rub some vegetable oil all over the baby's buttocks and genitals soon after birth (before the meconium appears). It will make cleaning off the meconium easier.

Over the next few days, the baby's bowel movements will change from black to green to yellow and will become very runny. After the first few days, the baby may have a bowel movement almost every time she eats, and should have at least four per day. This is a good sign that she is getting enough to eat.

Bathing the Baby

The baby will have a bath within the first couple of days. Unless the mother is accustomed to bathing newborns, the nurse or midwife will probably give the bath, teaching the mother at the same time. The usual advice is to give sponge baths until the dried cord falls off, but research suggests immersing a newborn in water is more comfortable for the baby and causes no harm. You can watch or help with the bath.

Caring for the Cord

The cord stump needs to be kept clean and dry. Arrange the baby's diaper so that it does not touch the cord. Clean the cord with water. The nurse or midwife will show you how to do this. The cord clamp is removed by the nurse or midwife, usually on the second day, leaving a black, dry stump that remains for a week or two and then drops off. The cord usually has a faintly foul smell, but call the baby's doctor if pus or red blood oozes from it.

Feeding the Baby

Breastfed babies need nothing but colostrum (the first "milk" to come from the breasts) and breast milk. They do not need formula, water, or glucose water unless they have low blood sugar. It is a good idea to begin breastfeeding as soon after birth as the baby is interested. Formula-fed babies should begin receiving formula when they seem ready to suck and when their condition is stable.

For more information about your role in feeding the baby, see "Getting Started with Breastfeeding," page 301.

Circumcision

If the baby is going to be circumcised, the procedure will be done in the hospital on the second day after birth, or, in the Jewish tradition, in the home or synagogue on the eighth day. In this procedure the foreskin is surgically removed from the end of the penis, or glans. Circumcision is usually, though not always, performed with anesthesia.

Purposes of Circumcision. The surgery is done

- To change the appearance of the penis to match the parents' preferences.
- To observe Jewish or other religious custom.
- To reduce the need for careful washing later in life.

Although no clear health benefits are attributable to routine circumcision of the newborn, many parents still choose it for their baby boys. The American Academy of Pediatrics does not recommend routine nonreligious circumcision of the newborn, but advises that parents become informed about the subject.

Disadvantages of Circumcision. Circumcision carries the same risks as all surgery: infection, hemorrhage, adhesions, pain, and human error.

- The procedure is clearly very painful. A local anesthetic is usually injected near or in the penis to reduce the pain of the procedure.
- Infection or hemorrhage occurs in about 1 in every 200 circumcisions. These conditions can usually be well controlled with medications and extra time in the hospital.
- There is a small possibility, especially with an inexperienced, unsupervised doctor, that the surgery will be done poorly— too much or too little foreskin may be removed.
- The circumcised penis usually takes seven to ten days to heal. Parents are taught how to take special care of the penis during this time, to avoid wet diapers and other irritations, and to observe the penis for signs of poor healing.
- If the newborn child is ill or if his penis is abnormal in structure, circumcision may be very harmful.

The popularity of this surgery has declined in the United States. The incidence of circumcision is now estimated at less than 60 percent, down from 85 percent in 1980.

Alternatives to Consider. You and the mother can

- Leave the baby uncircumcised. If you do, learn proper care of the uncircumcised penis (see "Recommended Resources"). Teach the child proper hygiene; washing the penis is about as complex as washing the ears.

- If you decide to have the baby circumcised, request anesthesia for the procedure, and, if possible, remain with the baby to comfort him.
- Leave the decision for the child to make himself when he reaches adulthood.

Baby-Care Skills

Many good videos, books, and classes are available on baby care and feeding (see "Recommended Resources"). The nurse or the midwife can also teach you and the mother many of the baby-care skills you need, such as

- Bathing the baby.
- Caring for the cord.
- Changing the baby's diapers.
- Positioning the baby for feeding.
- Feeding the baby (techniques).
- Burping the baby.
- Soothing a fussy baby.
- Caring for the baby's genitals.

The Next Few Days for the Mother

For the mother, the early postpartum period is marked by fatigue, emotional highs and lows, preoccupation with the baby, some pain, and an array of physical changes that affect most parts of her body.

She may be tired and excited at the same time, finding it difficult to sleep, but unable to exert herself very much without feeling worn out. A shower or a short walk is enough to send her straight back to bed.

The mother may be surprised by the variety of physical changes she experiences; these physical changes will require more attention than she ever expected.

Her Uterus

The nurse or midwife and the mother herself should check the uterus frequently in the first few days to be sure it remains contracted (see page 276). Remind the mother to continue doing this.

Afterpains

Especially if she has had a child before, the mother will feel afterpains, which can be quite intense, when the baby suckles or when the uterus contracts. Remind her to use her relaxation and breathing techniques. Pain medications are available if afterpains are severe. Afterpains go away in a few days.

Vaginal Discharge

The mother will have a vaginal discharge, called *lochia*, which is similar to a menstrual period. It starts out as a heavy red flow containing some clots, and gradually diminishes; it lasts from two to six weeks. If the lochia suddenly increases or if the mother passes large, golf-ball-sized clots, call her caregiver, because she may be bleeding from a blood vessel at the former site of the placenta.

The Perineum

After a vaginal birth, the mother's perineum will be sore, especially if she has had stitches. In any case, she may have swelling and bruising. You can suggest the following comfort measures:

- Applying an ice pack helps, especially during the first 24 hours.
- Sitting in a bath of warm water (a sitz bath) for 20 minutes, two or three times a day, is soothing. She should not wash in this water; it should be kept clean.
- Carefully patting her perineum dry (starting at the front, and moving toward the anus) or squirting it with warm water from a bottle after urinating or having a bowel movement is less irritating than wiping with toilet paper.
- Applying witch hazel–soaked pads to stitches and hemorrhoids is soothing.
- Doing the pelvic floor contraction exercise ("super-Kegel") promotes healing, reduces swelling, and restores strength. The mother tightens the muscles around her vagina and urethra

as she would if she were trying to hold back urine (see page 20). She should try to do 10 to 20 super-Kegels per day, and she should always do one as she sits down. She may find she cannot hold the super-Kegel for a full 20 seconds at first, but her ability will steadily improve.

Elimination

You may be surprised at how preoccupied the mother becomes with bowel movements and urination. These functions are more difficult than usual because her perineum is sore, her abdominal muscles are temporarily weak, her food and fluid intake have been interrupted by labor, and, now that it is no longer crowded by the baby, her bladder has an increased capacity.

If she is unable to urinate, even with all the tricks (running a faucet, urinating in the bath or shower, and so forth), she may have to have a catheter placed in her bladder to empty it. This is unpleasant, but it is better than letting her bladder become distended.

To help the mother avoid or reduce difficulties with the first bowel movement after giving birth, remind her to eat and drink high-fiber foods: prune juice, other juices, raw fruits and vegetables, bran breads or cereals, and so forth. Bulk-producing laxatives may also help. In addition, she might support her sore perineum by pressing toilet paper against it as she has a bowel movement. These measures also help if a woman has painful hemorrhoids.

Pain Following Cesarean Delivery

Post-cesarean pain results from the incision, from the stitches or clamps closing it, and from gas that commonly builds up in the mother's abdomen after this surgery. Activities such as turning over, getting out of bed, walking, and nursing the baby are usually very painful for a few days, but they hasten recovery. Help as much as you can to make these activities easier for her, by giving her a hand as she gets out of bed, offering a supportive arm as she walks, providing a pillow for her lap as she nurses the baby. The mother will gradually begin feeling better each day.

Clamps or stitches are removed on the second or third day

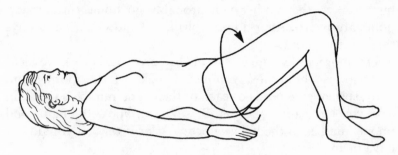

To reduce pain when rolling from her back to her side, the mother who has had a cesarean should raise and twist her hips before turning her shoulders.

after the delivery. The procedure is not very painful, and the pain from the incision will then decrease.

To help her reduce abdominal pain, encourage the mother to do the following:

- When rolling from her back to her side, she should first bend her knees so that her feet are flat on the bed. Then she should raise her hips, twist them to one side, and roll her shoulders to the side. This is much easier and far less painful than rolling over the usual way.
- She should avoid gas-producing foods (lentils and beans, foods in the cabbage family, cold or carbonated beverages).
- Before getting out of bed the first few times, she should warm up by doing an ankle-circling exercise and by raising her arms above her head several times.
- When holding the baby on her lap, she should place a pillow over the incision to protect it.
- She should ask the nurse to show her other ways to hold the baby to avoid pressure on her incision.

On Your Own at Home

Check the mother's insurance plan ahead of time to learn what to expect and what options she has after the birth. The usual hospital stay after a normal vaginal birth is 24 to 48 hours; after a cesarean, 72 to 96 hours. If the birth takes place in a birth center, the mother will probably go home three to six hours afterward. After a home birth, the midwife usually stays three to four hours.

The mother's caregiver should be sure you both have clear instructions about observations to make of the mother and baby, special care needs of each of them, and numbers to call in case you have any concerns. Be sure you know the name and phone number of the baby's doctor. Ask for these if you do not have them.

A follow-up appointment should be scheduled within the first week (preferably three or four days) after birth to check on breastfeeding and on the mother's and baby's health and well-being. If the baby was born at home, the midwife may make two or more home visits within the first several days.

Homecoming

Before the mother and the baby come home, take a moment to think about what they are coming home to. Is the house a mess? Is the sink full of dishes? Is the bed unmade? Is the baby's place (basket, box, crib, changing area) ready? There is nothing more disheartening for the mother than returning home to chaos. You want her to feel glad to get home, so try to provide a pleasant homecoming.

Prepare the home (it would be lovely if friends or family could help with this):

- Make the bed with fresh linens.
- Tidy up the house, do the dishes, and so forth.
- Make sure good food is available.
- Have a stack of fresh diapers ready (call a diaper service or buy some).
- Have a few welcoming touches around the house—fresh flowers, a "Welcome Home" poster.

Prepare for the ride home:

- Install the infant car seat (see page 16).
- Tidy up the inside of the car.

- Have enough gas so that you don't have to stop on the way home.
- Make sure the mother and the baby have clothes to wear home and that the baby has a blanket or two.
- Ask visitors not to come until at least the next day.

When the mother and the baby arrive home, you may all feel like celebrating. And with good reason! When you bring the baby home, you're introducing him to his own new world. The mother, too, may feel she has been away a long time and may be relieved to be in familiar surroundings once again. She has been through a lot and, unfortunately, fatigue will set in very soon. Perhaps the best thing for her to do is get into bed, snuggle with her loved ones, and bask in the warm feelings.

After a Home Birth

If the baby was born at home, there is probably a big cleanup operation ahead—dishes, lots of laundry, lots of trash, a bed to make with fresh linens. Sometimes everyone leaves soon after the birth, wanting to give the new family some quiet time together. And you are left with a huge cleanup project. Plan in advance, so you can avoid this situation:

- Ask the caregiver about cleanup ahead of time: (1) How much does she or he do? (2) What will need to be done? (3) What happens to the placenta? Sometimes the caregiver takes it and disposes of it. Some families bury it and plant a tree or a bush over it.
- Have large trash bags available during labor—one for disposable trash, one for laundry. As items are used, they can go right into the appropriate bags.
- If there are extra people available, assign ongoing and after-birth cleanup tasks: picking up and washing dishes, putting food away, doing laundry, taking trash out, straightening up the house.

Getting Help and Advice

The two of you will have your hands full, maintaining the household, feeding yourselves, and getting to know and care for the new family member, especially since all these tasks must be carried out in the midst of disrupted sleep schedules and the mother's postpartum adjustments. The brightest spot in all this is the deep and overwhelming love you feel toward your baby. The baby certainly makes it all worthwhile, but is there anything that could also make it a bit easier? The answer is yes: help.

Accept any and all offers of help from family and friends. Errand running, meal preparation, phone calls, housework—all these can be done by someone else. The best kind of help, however, is availability whenever you need it—day or night. Getting such help may not be possible unless you are fortunate enough to have a relative or close friend who can fit comfortably into the chaos. If the baby's grandmother or aunt comes to stay for a week or two, she can keep things running smoothly and offer some advice on questions about the baby. You will want to be sure this person is fostering the mother's self-confidence in meeting her baby's needs. This is no time for mother-daughter strife to rear its ugly head.

One way to ensure harmony is to invite the person most preferred by the mother, and to plan the visit for when the mother would prefer it—perhaps immediately after the birth, perhaps two to three weeks later. It also makes sense to spell out what you think you need from this person: "We are going to need help with running the household and cooking, because Jane gets really upset when the place gets messy. Knowing her, she'll run herself ragged trying to do everything even though the most important things are for her to spend lots of time with the baby, to get a good start with breastfeeding, and to get plenty of rest. Will you come and help us, so that she can devote herself to being a mother?"

Postpartum doulas are another solution to the problem of new family adjustment. These trained women can be hired for blocks of several hours per day for a period of a week or many weeks. See page 34 for more on postpartum doulas, and check "Recommended Resources" to locate one.

The Mother's Postpartum Emotions

During the early postpartum period the mother's emotions are changeable and unpredictable. One moment she may be rapturous and full of energy; the next, tired, frustrated, and in tears. The sudden changes in hormone production and body functions—as she goes from supporting the growth of a fetus during pregnancy to expelling a baby to resuming a nonpregnant state—take an emotional toll. Add to that her inevitable fatigue from loss of sleep during labor and during the first few days after the birth, as well as the stress of a profound role change, and it is not surprising that she is volatile.

If you are the mother's life partner as well as her birth partner, you have your own share of emotional adjustments—the role change to parenthood, your own fatigue, and a complete disruption in lifestyle. Even if you are a relative or a friend helping out temporarily, you are probably tired from the birth experience and from the strain of caring for the mother and the new baby.

As two tired people with a great many needs, you will be sustained through this stressful time by your underlying feelings for each other and by the joy and commitment you share in having a new baby. It helps to know that this situation *will* get better. Following are suggestions for getting through the emotional ups and downs of the first few days after the baby is born.

Postpartum Blues

If the mother seems sad or cries a lot, you may be surprised if this is not her usual style; you may feel helpless or guilty, believing that you are to blame or that it is up to you to make it right; you may worry about her; you may feel angry with her; or you may wonder if this situation is going to be permanent.

What Can You Do About Postpartum Blues? Here are some suggestions:

- First of all, let the mother cry. She does not have to have a reason. She needs to be able to cry without you (and everyone else) feeling you must help her get over it. Accept her need to cry with patience, tenderness, and empathy.

- Do not blame yourself. You almost certainly did not do anything to make her cry.
- Know that almost every woman sheds tears and goes on an emotional roller coaster for a few days; emotions are close to the surface after childbirth.
- Realize that this will probably pass after a few days. Give her time. Encourage her to nap and to rest (see "How to Get Enough Sleep," page 297).
- Ask her friends and relatives, especially those who have had children, to visit.
- Feel free to call the mother's caregiver, childbirth educator, or lactation consultant if you are worried about her.
- Look into mothers' groups or postpartum classes. They are becoming very popular as places where these feelings can be shared openly and discussed.

On rare occasions these blue feelings predominate and last for weeks. If you think this is happening, or if you feel under undue pressure, the mother may have postpartum depression or another mood disorder. Discuss your concerns with the mother, and call the resource people already mentioned. Ask the mother to go over "Unhappiness After Childbirth: A Self-Assessment" (page 295) with you, as a way to clarify her feelings. A referral from the mother's caregiver to a social worker, psychologist, or psychiatrist for counseling or therapy may be appropriate and very helpful. A complete physical exam, with blood tests to check levels of various hormones, might reveal a physical condition that could be contributing to depression. Or a support group alone might help the mother recover from her depressed feelings. Consider these options if the mother is predominantly depressed after a few weeks.

Practical Matters at Home

Much of the turmoil of the postpartum period can be avoided if you're prepared for it in advance and if you can simplify your lives for a while. Whether you are the mother's life partner or a

UNHAPPINESS AFTER CHILDBIRTH: A SELF-ASSESSMENT

Circle the answer that comes closest to how you have felt *in the past seven days*, not just how you feel today.

1. I have been able to laugh and see the funny side of things . . .
   a. As much as I always could.   b. Not quite as much as I used to.
   c. Definitely not as much as I used to.   d. Not at all.
2. I have looked forward with enjoyment to things . . .
   a. As much as I always did.   b. Not quite as much as I used to.
   c. Definitely not as much as I used to.   d. Not at all.
3. I have blamed myself unnecessarily when things went wrong . . .
   a. Not at all.   b. Very little.   c. Some of the time.
   d. Most of the time.
4. I have been anxious or worried for no good reason . . .
   a. Not at all.   b. Very little.   c. Some of the time.
   d. Most of the time.
5. I have felt scared or panicked for no good reason . . .
   a. Not at all.   b. Very little.   c. Some of the time.
   d. Most of the time.
6. I have been feeling overwhelmed . . .
   a. Not at all; I've been coping very well.
   b. Very little; I've been coping pretty well.
   c. Some of the time; I haven't been coping as well as usual.
   d. Quite a lot; I haven't been able to cope at all.
7. I have been so unhappy that I've had difficulty sleeping . . .
   a. Not at all.   b. Very little.   c. Some of the time.
   d. Most of the time.
8. I have felt sad or miserable . . .
   a. Not at all.   b. Very little.   c. Some of the time.
   d. Most of the time.
9. I have been so unhappy that I've been crying . . .
   a. Not at all.   b. Very little.   c. Some of the time.
   d. Most of the time.
10. The thought of harming myself or my baby has occurred to me . . .
    a. Not at all.   b. Very little.   c. Some of the time.
    d. Most of the time.

If you have a feeling after completing this form that something isn't right, or if you have any questions about your emotional well-being, please contact your childbirth educator, doula, doctor or midwife, or a mental-health therapist.

Adapted from J. L. Cox and J. M. Holden, "Detection of Postnatal Depression: Development of the 10-Item Edinburgh Postnatal Depression Scale," *British Journal of Psychiatry* 150 (1987): 782–86.

relative or friend helping out, the following suggestions will help all of you get through these first days until the household becomes more settled.

Fatigue and Sleep Deprivation

The mother is tired. You may be tired, too. If after being her birth partner you are now her "at home" support person, you are probably running out of energy yourself. Sleep deprivation is a serious problem among new parents that is often ignored. It may cause inadequate milk supply; severe mood swings (including postpartum emotional disorders); and inability to deal with the baby's crying, other minor annoyances, and even simple decision making (about what to have for dinner, for instance). Fatigue makes *everything* worse, and adequate rest makes *everything* better—the mother's appetite, her feelings toward the baby and toward you, her mood, her milk supply, her patience, and so on.

And yet people simply resign themselves to the belief that all new parents, especially mothers, cannot possibly get enough sleep. This is not true. It is possible for most new mothers to get enough sleep. To do so, however, they must give sleep a very high priority (right next to being sure the baby is fed and cared for), and restructure their lives to ensure they get enough. It does not work for the mother to simply "sleep when the baby sleeps," as most women are advised to do. If the baby is often wide awake when the mother needs to sleep, you might help out by looking after the baby.

Until things have settled into a comfortable routine, give a high priority to getting enough sleep. Unplug the phone, and keep a "Do Not Disturb" sign on the front door until one of you is ready to get up.

Fussy, Crying Baby

Entire books have been written about fussy babies (see "Recommended Resources"). In the first few days, a fussy baby can usually be soothed by

- Feeding or burping.
- Changing her diaper.

HOW TO GET ENOUGH SLEEP

(This applies to both parents until the breadwinner returns to employment. Then he or she will have to get more sleep at night and less during the day.)

Recall how many hours of daily sleep you needed before pregnancy in order to function well. Six hours? Eight hours? That is the amount of sleep you now owe yourself every day.

Since you cannot get this amount of sleep in one stretch, because of interruptions for feedings and baby care, you will require more hours in bed to get your allotted amount of sleep. Plan to stay in bed or keep going back to bed until you have slept your allotted number of hours. This means that except for meals and trips to the bathroom, you do not get up in the early morning. Keep a mental note of approximately how much time you have slept at each stretch, and stay in your nightclothes until you have slept the required number of hours. You may have to stay in bed from ten at night until noon the next day to get eight hours of sleep! If that's what it takes, do it. Then brush your teeth, take a shower, and dress.

Many parents find it easier to follow this advice if the baby sleeps with them or nearby.

As your baby grows and begins to sleep for longer stretches, it will take you less time to get enough sleep.

- Letting the baby suck on your (clean) little finger: place your finger in her mouth with the nail down on her tongue and the soft pad touching the roof of her mouth. She might take your finger more eagerly at first if you wet it.
- Swaddling the baby snugly in a blanket.
- Picking her up, rocking or walking her, or changing her position in bed. "Wear" the baby by carrying her close to your body in a baby carrier or sling.
- Holding the baby against your shoulder while bouncing on a birth ball. This works wonders.
- Creating "white noise"—the sounds of a dishwasher or a washing machine; peaceful recorded music; or, best of all, lullabies crooned in the baby's ear.

Don't leave a tiny baby crying. The first few days after birth are a major adjustment for the baby, too. A newborn needs the comfort and security of feeling your bodies and hearing your voices nearby. Do not worry about spoiling the baby: You cannot spoil her by meeting her basic needs.

Scheduling the Baby's Sleeping and Feeding

Don't even try to get the baby on a schedule in the first few weeks. Instead, discover the baby's own schedule, and pattern your life around that. Focus on meeting the baby's needs; try to figure out how he tells you he is hungry, curious, interested, bored, uncomfortable, or overstimulated. Let the baby call the shots. It is much easier for the household to adjust to the baby at first than to make the baby adjust to the household. Make it your goal to meet the baby's needs, as expressed by the baby—you will all be happier if you do. Read *Your Amazing Newborn* (see "Recommended Resources") to help you understand the baby.

Meals

Time for meal preparation hardly exists during the busy first days at home, yet good food, quickly available, is a must. Try the following:

- *Prepare meals in advance.* Before the birth, prepare a few dishes—such as soups, casseroles, and stews—that will either keep for several days or will freeze.
- *Purchase quick, nutritious, tasty foods.* Foods that need little or no preparation—that you can grab and eat—are good choices for the first few weeks. Such foods include yogurt, fruit, granola and nuts, cottage cheese, hard cheese, raw vegetables, and whole-grain breads and crackers. Try to have these on hand before the birth so you won't have to go shopping right away. This is the time, too, to search the deli counter at the grocery store for nourishing, delicious prepared food.
- *Fix dishes that last for a while.* For example, you can roast a turkey and pick from it for a week; or wash, cut, and chill raw vegetables to keep in the refrigerator for munching.

- *Accept food from friends and relatives.* If people ask how they can help, tell them you'd love a main dish.
- *Remember the mother's dietary needs.* Her postpartum diet should be as good as her pregnancy diet was. If she is breast-feeding, she will need 200 to 300 calories more than normal each day. She will also need at least two quarts of liquids each day.

Household Chores

The first few days at home are busy and full of adjustments. Do the mother and yourself a big favor: If you have no help, plan to do the minimum in the way of household chores—just enough to maintain sanity. It may be easier if you have "super-cleaned" before the baby was born; if you haven't, just close your eyes and let things accumulate for a while. Simplify your lives so you are free to care for and enjoy the baby and to get enough rest.

11

Getting Started with Breastfeeding

Your role when the mother breastfeeds may seem unclear, because it is not as simple as taking over the feeding for her when she is tired. It is more a matter of supporting her decision to breastfeed and helping simplify her life while she does it. It really helps if you have some knowledge and conviction about the advantages of breastfeeding.

Advantages of Breastfeeding

The advantages of breastfeeding are many, for everyone involved. For the family,

- It costs much less to breastfeed than to formula-feed.
- Formula preparation and bottle washing chores are avoided.

For the mother,

- Breastfeeding hastens her uterus's return to normal by causing it to contract with every feeding.
- Hormones associated with breastfeeding cause relaxation and feelings of contentment.

- Once the initial learning period has passed, most women find breastfeeding very satisfying.

For the baby,

- Breast milk is perfectly suited to the baby's nutritional requirements.
- Breast milk contains substances (immunoglobulins and antibodies from the mother) that provide important protection against illness.
- Breast milk changes in composition as the baby grows and his nutritional requirements change.
- Problems with allergies, indigestion, and overfeeding are fewer with breast milk than with formula.
- The milk is always at the right temperature and instantly available.
- Long-term advantages of superior jaw development, reduced likelihood of obesity, and better ability to handle dietary fats are also attributed to breastfeeding.

Because of all these advantages, most mothers today decide to breastfeed. There are challenges to overcome, however, before breastfeeding becomes easy, quick, and convenient. A lack of experience may lead parents to doubt whether the baby is getting enough milk, to worry that the baby nurses too often or not enough. They may not feel they can trust the process.

There is much to know to get off to a good start with breastfeeding. Before the baby is born, identify helpful resources:

- A good breastfeeding book can be a godsend in the middle of the night! (See "Recommended Resources.")
- Most hospitals have lactation consultants, but they may not be available for ongoing support. The baby's doctor or your childbirth educator can probably refer you to a lactation consultant who can provide later or longer-term help.
- Support groups such as La Leche League are listed under "Breastfeeding" in the white, business, or yellow pages of the phone book.
- The baby's doctor will help her know if her baby is thriving on breast milk and can suggest helpful resources.
- Friends who have breastfed can advise on helpful products

and resources, and can empathize and assist with problems.
- Internet websites provide products and information, and news groups offer advice and support.
- Videotapes are available that teach and illustrate basic principles (see "Recommended Resources").

Make a list of names, phone numbers, and addresses of all these helpful resources. Post it on the mother's refrigerator.

You should also both take a breastfeeding class to learn the basics. Most organizations and hospitals offering childbirth classes also offer breastfeeding classes.

A supportive partner is a nursing woman's best resource, even if the partner does not know very much about breastfeeding. Your belief that the mother can do it and your help are crucial: being that extra pair of hands to help position the baby for feeding; keeping her fed and as rested as she can be; changing diapers; bathing, soothing, rocking, or bouncing the baby; taking the baby for short walks or rides outside (depending on the weather); being patient and loving through the early adjustments.

Getting Off to a Good Start

A good start with breastfeeding depends on

- Frequent feeding of the baby on cue (whenever the baby gives indications that he wants the breast), beginning as soon after birth as the baby will suckle.
- Recognition of the baby's feeding cues. A baby usually indicates her desire for the breast long before she cries from hunger. Here are some feeding clues:
  - Bringing a hand to her mouth.
  - Opening her mouth and turning her head toward anything that brushes her cheek ("rooting").
  - Making sucking sounds and motions with her mouth and tongue.
  - Fussing.
  - Sucking avidly on a finger placed in her mouth.
- A good "latch" between the baby's mouth and the breast.
- Availability of advice from a lactation consultant or other knowledgeable person.

- *Your* help and positive support.
- Freedom from excessive difficulty.

I mention the last item because, on rare occasions, a woman who wants very much to breastfeed has one problem after another, even when working closely with a breastfeeding counselor. If breastfeeding is the way most of her friends and family choose to feed their babies, a woman may feel a great deal of pressure to do the same. If she finally gives up in exasperation and disappointment, she may feel depressed, uncertain, and ashamed over her decision. But only she can balance the advantages and disadvantages of her situation. She should get the best support and advice available, and if feeding problems are still insurmountable, she is correct to formula-feed. And she should be forgiving of herself.

Your understanding and support of her decision will help her immensely. Most important, try to deal with overzealous advocates of breastfeeding who may not understand that the mother has made her best effort to breastfeed. Such people sometimes become judgmental, and increase a woman's guilt and disappointment.

Early Concerns

Breastfeeding does not come easily at first to most women. It takes two to four weeks to reach the point where all the mother has to do is put the baby near her breast to get him to latch on and suckle. In the meantime, problems such as temporary nipple soreness, lack of sleep, and concern over milk supply have to be overcome. Both you and the mother need information and guidelines on what is normal and how to solve these problems. The resources you have lined up (see page 302) will help with these concerns.

Milk Supply

How can you know if the mother is making enough milk? If the baby needs to nurse frequently, does it mean the mother is not making enough milk to satisfy the baby's hunger? It sometimes is difficult to trust such an imprecise process as breastfeeding. These facts may help:

- The mother makes a very small quantity of colostrum for the first two to four days after birth. It is enough to satisfy all the baby's nutritional requirements for the first few days.
- The colostrum is replaced by milk on the third or fourth day after birth. The frequency and total amount of time spent suckling help determine when the milk "comes in" and how much milk the mother makes.
- Young babies normally nurse often—8 to 18 times a day. This may come as a surprise to the mother, who will spend many hours every day breastfeeding. Generally, the more a baby suckles, the more milk the mother makes.
- Babies do not nurse at regular intervals; they "bunch up" several feedings in a row, and then go without feeding for a relatively long stretch. It is normal for a baby to nurse four times in six hours, then sleep for three to four hours before the next feeding.
- An ample milk supply is indicated by these signs: how the breasts feel (more heavy and full before a feeding than afterward); whether milk can be expressed or drips from the breasts; whether the baby is wetting her diapers and having bowel movements (after the milk comes in, six to eight wet diapers and four or more bowel movements a day are good signs for the first four weeks); and whether the baby noticeably swallows after every few sucks. Weight gain is a clear sign that the baby is getting enough milk, although the baby may not begin to gain until he is a few days old.

If the baby appears not to be getting enough milk, try the 24-Hour Cure (page 309).

Fatigue and Lack of Sleep in the Mother

Because young babies nurse frequently and sometimes fuss during the night, long stretches of sleep are no longer possible for the mother, or for you if you're trying to help at night. Sleep tends to come in the form of two- to three-hour naps between feedings. This normal change in sleep patterns is not a major problem if you and the mother can catch up with a nap or two.

If not, fatigue sets in, and it interferes with all aspects of parenting and daily living. Follow the instructions on page 297.

The mother may get more sleep, and the baby may fuss less, if she nurses him in bed at night and naps or sleeps with or near him. This way she can doze as she feeds the baby and does not have to get up as much. But if the mother is uncomfortable having the baby in bed with her, this solution will not work. If fatigue becomes a major concern for the mother, try the 24-Hour Cure (page 309).

Breast and Nipple Pain

Breast pain in the first few days may be caused by

Engorgement. Breast milk replaces colostrum after one and a half to four days. It usually "comes in" over a period of eight to twelve hours. Some women's breasts become extremely full and painful, or engorged, making it difficult for the baby to latch on. Frequent breastfeeding helps to prevent severe engorgement, but the baby's appetite and ability at the breast may not match the milk supply at first. If the breasts are too firm to allow the baby to get a good latch, the mother should soften them as follows: She should express a small amount of milk before she feeds the baby, either by hand or with a mechanical pump. She can apply hot packs or let the shower run over her breasts to start the flow of milk. Engorgement subsides after a few days, when a balance is reached between the amount of milk needed by the baby and the amount produced by the mother.

Engorgement sometimes occurs even in women who do not breastfeed, but a lack of suckling and a pressure binder (an elastic bandage wrapped around the chest to flatten the breasts) will stop milk production.

Nipple pain may be caused by

Prolonged, Vigorous Suckling. Some babies suck harder and longer than others. Early nipple soreness may be greater with such babies, but it passes within a week or so if the latch (the connection between mouth and breast) is good. It is considered within normal limits if soreness occurs each time the baby latches but then subsides after about a minute of suckling, and the rest of the feeding is comfortable. If soreness persists throughout a feeding, it may be because of a poor latch (see below).

Trying to limit the baby's suckling time to 3 or 5 minutes does not reduce soreness and is unnecessary. If the baby's suckling is very prolonged, however, the mother could try switching breasts after 15 minutes of steady suckling. The most important thing is to check the baby's latch (see below).

It is important not to fall into the trap of giving a bottle to "rest" the breasts, unless the soreness is extreme. In this case, the mother should regularly pump her milk to keep up her supply, and she should seek help from a professional lactation consultant.

Thrush. A yeast infection in the baby's mouth can spread to the mother's nipples, causing deep, severe pain during nursing. If the mother has this kind of pain, check the baby's mouth for patches of white film on his gums, his tongue, or the roof of his mouth. Check the mother's nipples as well for irritated or whitish patches. A thrush infection is most likely to occur if the mother or the baby has recently taken antibiotics or if the mother is prone to yeast infections. Call the baby's doctor if you suspect thrush.

A Poor Latch. Improper suckling may cause the mother excessive nipple soreness. If the baby nibbles or "clicks" (breaks the suction with each suck), the mother's nipples will hurt more than is normally expected. Her nurse or midwife, a lactation consultant, her childbirth educator, or a good book on breastfeeding (see "Recommended Resources") can help with the latch.

A good latch means the baby is positioned correctly and her mouth takes in a large amount of *areola* (the dark circle around the nipple). When held in the mother's arms, the baby should lie on her side ("tummy to tummy") rather than on her back. Other good positions are lying side by side and the "football" or "clutch" hold, in which the mother sits up, holding the baby beside and facing her. The baby's feet are behind the mother, and the baby's head is held by the mother at her breast. In all positions, ordinary pillows, or the now popular horseshoe-shaped nursing pillows, are useful for propping the mother and the baby comfortably. In all positions, too, the baby's face is held very close to the breast, with her nose touching it, so she doesn't pull hard on the nipple with every suck. Her mouth should open wide as she latches on to the breast.

Treating Sore Nipples. The mother can treat nipple soreness in the following ways:

- Rub a little colostrum or milk into the nipples and allow them to dry.
- Dry the nipples after each feeding with a hair dryer (on its lowest setting) held at arm's length. This feels wonderful, and thoroughly dries the nipples.
- Apply ice to the nipples just before a feeding to reduce sensation.
- Soak black (not herbal) tea bags in warm water, place them on the nipples, and cover the tea bags with plastic wrap. The mother should lie on her back with the tea bags in place for about 10 minutes two or three times a day. Tea contains a small amount of tannic acid, which seems to toughen skin.
- Rub unscented purified hydrous lanolin into the nipples (unless she is allergic to wool).
- Avoid washing the nipples with soap, even if they are protected by a coating of lanolin. Soap makes soreness worse. Rinsing with water is sufficient for cleanliness.
- Expose the breasts to the air by lowering the flaps of her bra, or by wearing no bra.
- Begin each nursing on the less sore side.
- Reduce suckling time to 15 minutes per side until the soreness begins to subside.
- If the soreness is extreme and the nipples are bleeding, stop breastfeeding, and pump milk for a day or so to get healing started. During this time, give the baby pumped breast milk or formula from a bottle.
- Try breast shields, thin silicone nipple covers with holes that allow the milk to flow out. They may protect the nipples from further damage during nursings.
- Take acetaminophen, not aspirin or ibuprofen, if she needs pain medications.

If these measures fail, consult a lactation consultant, child-birth educator, the baby's physician, or a good book on breast-feeding (see "Recommended Resources").

The 24-Hour Cure

During the first few weeks after birth, the mother and baby are mastering the art of breastfeeding. The 24-Hour Cure can solve some of the problems that arise, such as the following:

- Doubts about whether the mother is making enough milk.
- Fatigue, lack of sleep, or anxiety in the mother.
- Lack of appetite, poor nourishment, or low fluid intake in the mother.
- Slow weight gain or weight loss in the baby.
- "Nipple confusion"—that is, the baby seems to prefer a rubber nipple or nipple shield to the mother's breast.

The cure promotes frequent, efficient suckling and an abundant milk supply by nurturing both the mother and the baby. The mother gets complete rest, plenty of good food and drink, and freedom from all responsibility other than feeding and cuddling her baby. The baby gets prolonged skin-to-skin contact with the mother and constant access to her breast and nurturance.

Here is how to do the cure:

- Set aside a full 24 hours when the mother can have your help. Use your day off, or get a friend or relative to take your place. Around-the-clock help is essential.
- Make sure the mother does not have sore, blistered, or cracked nipples when she begins the cure. The causes of the soreness need to be addressed before starting the cure (see "Treating Sore Nipples," page 308).
- The mother goes to bed with the baby. They both wear as little clothing as practical under the bedcovers so the baby can get lots of warm skin-to-skin contact, which will stimulate his suckling reflex and interest in feeding.
- The mother may read, watch TV, chat with you (no visitors, please), or, most important, doze. The extra sleep makes a big difference, even though it comes in short snatches.

- She gets out of bed *only to go to the bathroom*—not to eat, answer the phone, do housework, or anything else.
- Supply her with liquids; place water or juice within her reach. She should drink about two to three quarts of liquid during the 24 hours.
- Fix tasty, nutritious meals for her. Tempt her appetite with foods she is unlikely to prepare for herself. If she has been relying on take-out fast foods or cold ready-to-eat foods, she will love a hot, home-cooked meal or two.
- The baby should stay in bed with her, except when a diaper change is necessary, or when the baby is fussy (but not willing to nurse) and needs to be briefly walked or rocked. Then you should take care of the baby.
- Whenever the baby awakens or seems at all interested in suckling, the mother offers her breast. Do not give the baby a bottle of either formula or breast milk, unless he is seriously underweight (in this case you need to consult the baby's doctor, a lactation consultant, or a breastfeeding support organization such as La Leche League, which is listed in the white pages of the phone book).

The combination of rest and nourishment for the mother and skin-to-skin contact and unlimited suckling for the baby almost always results in a marked increase in the mother's milk production, improved suckling by the baby, and a much happier mother.

If the mother is unable to closely follow the 24-Hour Cure, or if it fails to solve the problem, consult the baby's doctor, a lactation consultant, or La Leche League.

When to Give the Baby a Bottle

Most babies need to be able to get milk from a bottle sooner or later. You may have heard stories about babies who won't take a bottle, and about how distraught the mother becomes when she needs the baby to do so. For a smooth introduction to bottle feeding, timing is crucial. Too-early bottle feeding may interfere with the baby's learning to breastfeed. But if the bottle is introduced too late, the baby may refuse it.

It is wise not to rush bottle feeding with a breastfed baby, for two reasons. First, while the baby is getting used to the human nipple, it may be confusing for him to suck from a rubber nipple. Different sucking techniques—different mouth and jaw motions—are required for human and rubber nipples. The baby may not be able to go from one to the other. (Of course, there are circumstances when a very young infant must be bottle-fed. A lactation consultant can be very helpful in teaching a baby who has been bottle-fed to suckle at the breast, when he is able to do so.)

Second, when a baby takes milk from a bottle, he spends less time suckling at the breast. This may slow milk production, because it is the suckling that stimulates the breasts to produce. A shortage of breast milk may result.

If you will need to feed the baby with a bottle at some time, wait until the baby regularly latches on and suckles at the breast easily, without coaxing, and until the milk supply is clearly plentiful. Most babies are good latchers and sucklers by three to four weeks of age (although some may need several more weeks). If the bottle is introduced at this time, the baby will probably adjust easily. You must continue to offer the bottle regularly after that, however—about twice a week—or you may have to struggle to get the baby to take a bottle later.

It is usually preferable that someone other than the mother give the bottle to the baby; he may insist on the mother's breast if she is right there. Feed the baby the mother's expressed milk, preferably, or formula.

If the baby is reluctant to take the bottle after becoming accustomed to the breast, allow a couple of weeks for the baby to learn to use the bottle before the mother leaves him for a significant length of time with you or a babysitter. With persistence on your part, the baby will eventually take the bottle. But if it ever happens that the mother is unavailable to nurse and the baby will not take the bottle, you can try squirting milk into a corner of his mouth with an eyedropper.

Once Breastfeeding Is Established

By two to six weeks of age, most babies and their mothers find breastfeeding to be a pleasant, quick, convenient method of feeding. Although there may still be some hurdles ahead, the greatest difficulties are behind most breastfeeding mothers and babies by this time, and the closeness and pleasure they share are most satisfying.

Parting Words

The family is launched. The baby is born and getting used to the world; the mother is no longer pregnant and is adjusting to being on constant call. Your job as birth partner is over. The excitement is over and you may feel strangely let down.

Now what? It will take a while to absorb and integrate all that has happened. This birth has transformed you into a parent, or grandparent, or more-special-than-ever friend. You will never be the same, and you will always treasure this experience.

Congratulations.

Recommended
Resources

Following is a list of publications, audio- and videotapes, and online resources that provide added information on pregnancy, birth, and parenting. Doris Olson, executive director of the International Childbirth Education Association, provided permission to use the descriptions of most of the books and tapes as they appear in *ICEA Bookmarks*, the catalog of the ICEA bookstore, where they may be purchased (ICEA, P.O. Box 20048, Minneapolis, MN 55420, phone: 800-624-4934 or fax: 952-854-8772). Most well-stocked bookstores also carry these books.

Pregnancy

Flanagan, Geraldine Lux. *Beginning Life*. DK Publishing, 1996. Tells the story of life from conception to birth through beautiful photographs and compelling narrative.

Heinowitz, Jack. *Pregnant Fathers*. Parents as Partners Press, 1995. A book for expectant fathers, covering such topics as hidden feelings and needs, communication, problem solving, participation in labor and birth, welcoming baby, and early parenthood.

Jiminéz, Sherry L.M. *The Pregnant Woman's Comfort Guide*. Avery Publishing Group, 1992. A handbook that provides the expectant mother with natural and effective treatments for more than 70 of the most common discomforts of pregnancy and the postpartum period.

Mungeam, Frank. *A Guy's Guide to Pregnancy*. Fine Communications, 1998. Written from a man's viewpoint to help men understand how pregnancy will affect them, their partner, and their relationship.

Stillerman, Elaine. *Mother Massage*. Delta, 1992. Provides techniques for relieving discomforts of pregnancy; designed to be used either alone or with a partner. Numerous types of massage are covered. Fully illustrated.

England, Pam, and Rob Horowitz. *Birthing from Within.* Partera Press, 1998. Includes information on the art of birthing, preparing the birth place, father and birth companions, and parenting. Illustrated

Freedman, Lois Halzel. *Birth as a Healing Experience.* Harrington Park Press, 1999. Emphasizes and examines the emotional aspects of pregnancy and postpartum. Focuses on the healing potential of pregnancy, childbirth, and postpartum rather than the medical aspects.

Goer, Henci. *The Thinking Woman's Guide to a Better Birth.* Perigee, 1999. Provides clear, concise information about issues surrounding cesareans, ultrasound, gestational diabetes, breech babies, inducing labor, IVs, electronic fetal monitoring, rupturing membranes, epidurals, episiotomies, vaginal birth after cesarean, and more.

Harper, Barbara. *Gentle Birth Choices.* Inner Traditions International Limited, 1994. Discusses alternatives available, including giving birth in a freestanding birth center, at home, or in a hospital birthing room. Offers advice to couples wishing to explore options of water birth.

Kitzinger, Sheila. *The Complete Book of Pregnancy and Childbirth,* New Edition. Knopf, 1996. Comprehensive guide to pregnancy and childbirth, fully illustrated with photographs, drawings, and diagrams.

Korte, Diana. *The VBAC Companion.* The Harvard Common Press, 1997. Helps women make the choice of having a vaginal birth after cesarean. Addresses mother's concerns and provides resources needed for giving birth the way she wishes.

Simkin, Penny, Janet Whalley, and Ann Keppler. *Pregnancy, Childbirth and the Newborn, Fourth Edition.* Meadowbrook Press, 2001. Covers nutrition, fetal development, prenatal procedures, health-care providers, birth places, birth plans, labor support techniques, medical interventions, exercises, relaxation, and breastfeeding, with strong presentation of parental choice and excellent charts.

Simkin, Penny. *Simkin's Rating of Comfort Measures for Childbirth.* Canadian Childbirth Teaching Aids, 1997. Uses Simkin's rating system to explain 18 different ways to relieve pain in labor. Each method is rated in seven areas. Includes a Comfort Measures Chart comparing all the methods.

Physical Conditioning for the Partner

Crunch Fitness Centers, *Get Fit in a Crunch.* Hatherleigh Press, 1999. A four-week workout plan to build strength and cardiovascular fitness in a program to fit a busy lifestyle.

De Lisle. *The Navy Seal Workout: the Complete Total-Body Fitness Program.* NTC/Contemporary Publishing, 1998. Provides a variety of exercises and techniques to improve total body strength and endurance. Exercises can be done in any setting.

Stillbirth/Miscarriage

Lothrop, Hannah. *Help, Comfort and Hope After Losing Your Baby in Pregnancy or the First Year.* Fisher Books, 1997. Speaks to those who have lost a child through miscarriage, stillbirth, neonatal death, sudden infant death, or termination of pregnancy. Also for caregivers who help parents through this difficult time.

Schwiebert, Pat, and Paul Kirk. *When Hello Means Goodbye.* Perinatal Loss, 1993. Basic reference for parents whose child dies, and for childbirth educators helping these parents.

Fathering

DeMorier, Everett. *Crib Notes for the First Year of Fatherhood.* Fairview Press, 1998. Written to save new fathers time, money, and energy, it provides practical advice on supporting the new mother, balancing work and family, etc.

Downey, Peter. *So You're Going to Be a Dad.* Fisher Books, 2000. A book about the trials and joys of parenting, written for dads with little or no knowledge or experience with parenting.

Goldman, Marcus Jacob, M.D. *The Joy of Fatherhood*. Prima Publishing, 2000. A dad-to-dad book; the author shares his insights and advice. Real-life experiences and thoughts from dads are shared throughout the book.

Infant Care and Feeding

Best, Judith. *How to Soothe and Amuse Your Baby From Birth to Three Months*. Remedios Publishing, 1995. Twenty-nine useful techniques are described for calming a fussy newborn and more than 60 playtime activities to stimulate growth and development.

Blocker, Ann K. *Baby Basics*. John Wiley & Sons, 1997. Filled with advice and useful tips, this book is written to help new parents make the best choices and most practical decisions for their child.

Huggins, Kathleen. *The Nursing Mother's Companion*, Fourth Edition. The Harvard Common Press, 1999. A practical, step-by-step guide to make breastfeeding easier, safer, and happier for mothers and babies. Addresses special needs: working mothers, cesarean mothers, mothers of twins, and mothers of premature or handicapped babies.

Karlin, Elyce Zorn, Diane Williams, and Daisy Spier. *The Complete African-American Baby Checklist*. William Morrow & Company, 1999. A guide for first-time black parents, enabling them to bring their baby into a happy, healthy home, free from stress and filled with love.

Klaus, Marshall, M.D., and Phyllis H. Klaus. *Your Amazing Newborn*. Perseus Press, 2000. Celebrates baby's extraordinary abilities during the first hours and days of life. Enhanced by more than 120 photographs, all of babies less than two weeks old.

Lansky, Vicki. *Baby Proofing Basics*. Book Peddlers, 1991. Offers simple, practical safety tips and information on available child safety products to help create a safe environment for children.

Leach, Penelope. *Your Baby and Child*. Knopf, Revised Edition, 1997. Comprehensive and sensitive guide to a child's first five years. Lavishly illustrated.

McClure, Vimala Schneider. *Infant Massage, Third Edition*. Bantam Books, 1989. Clearly illustrated guide to massaging your baby, including songs to sing and games to play.

Sears, William, and Martha Sears. *The Baby Book*. Little Brown & Company, 1993. Covers all the practical information on baby care, and helps parents fully understand their baby's emotional needs. Based on the parenting style called "attachment parenting."

Todd, Linda. *You and Your Newborn Baby*. The Harvard Common Press, 1993. A practical and sensitive guide to the mother's physical and emotional recovery after birth, from infant care to baby's early development.

Audiotape

Simkin, Penny. *Relax for Childbirth*. Narrated audiotape with music by Margaret Wakely Harris, 1988. This 16-minute tape begins with an original lullaby sung by Harris, expressing feelings toward the soon-to-be-born baby. The relaxation exercise emphasizes tension release and slow breathing and includes suggestions to prepare for birth.

Videotape

Benedict, Ines. *Infant Massage: The Power of Touch*. Video International Entertainment World, 1995. Multicultural class of moms receiving instruction on and demonstrating infant massage.

Johnson & Johnson Pediatric Institute Limited. *Amazing Talents of the Newborn*, 1998. This 30-minute program is designed to enhance appreciation for the innate and often overlooked abilities of the newborn, and in so doing to help broaden understanding of the newborn's developmental needs.

Simkin, Penny. *Comfort Measures for Childbirth with Penny Simkin*, 1996. Shows how to do all the comfort techniques taught by Penny Simkin.

Vida Health Communications, Incorporated. *Baby Basics*, 1987. Provides instruction, demonstration, and support to new and expectant parents, offering practical advice on the newborn, daily care, feeding methods, infant security, and more.

Online Resources for Parents-to-be

www.aap.org

The American Academy of Pediatrics website contains information on all aspects of infant and child health, including car seats, immunizations, well child care, and much more.

www.babycenter.com

Provides information on pregnancy, fetal development, labor and birth, and Dads' Zone. Includes live chats and message boards.

www.dona.org

Everything you need to know about doulas, and how to find and select the right doula for you.

www.firsttimedad.com

A resource just for fathers from pregnancy through early parenthood.

www.parentsplace.com

Provides information on infant/child development at all stages and support through message boards and live chats. Contains many articles by experts.

www.pennysimkin.com

The author's website contains information about birth and parenting, along with her speaking schedule and other activities.

Index

A

Abdominal lifting, 155
Abdominal pain, postpartum, 288-289
Abdominal stroking, 154-155
Active labor, 68-69
 birth partner's feelings during, 71
 birth partner's role in, 71-73, 90
 caregiver's role in, 70-71
 described, 90
 duration of, 69
 illustrated, 77
 mother's feelings during, 69-70
 pain in, 68
Acupressure
 as comfort measure, 126-127
 to stimulate labor, 150-151
Afterpains, 287
Amnioinfusion
 alternatives to, 189
 described, 188-189
 disadvantages of, 189
Amniotic fluid, examination of, 174
Analgesia
 defined, 228
 inhalation, 240
Anesthesia
 defined, 228
 epidural, 230, 231-232, 233-235, 241-243
 general, 229, 236, 245
 local, 228-229, 232-233, 235-236, 246-247
 regional, 230, 231-235, 241-244
 spinal, 230, 231-232, 233-235, 243-244

Apgar score, 174, 175
Areola, defined, 307
Aromatherapy, 129
Arrested labor, 210, 256
Artificial rupture of membranes (AROM)
 alternatives to, 188
 described, 187
 disadvantages of, 188
 indications for, 187-188, 190
 purposes of, 187
Atrial natriuretic factor (ANF), 119
Attention focusing, to alleviate pain, 104-105
Augmentation of labor, 189-195
 methods of, 189-190
 purposes of, 190-192

B

Baby. *See* Infant; Newborn
Backache
 causes of, 152-153
 comfort measures to ease, 158
 incidence of, 152
 as sign of labor, 46
 treatment and prevention of, 128, 129, 153-158
Bag of waters breakage
 premature, 48-49
 as sign of labor, 46, 47
Barbiturates, 238
Baths, 115
 modesty issues, 120
 to reduce pain and speed labor, 118-119
 safety of, 120-121
 timing of, 119
 water temperature for, 119-120
Bearing down, 73-74, 76